To Justin

Live in vision!

Bruce A. Tolle

#chuckstrong

For broadcast journalists, objectivity is vital. Every once in a while, though, objectivity, schmobjectivity. When Coach Pagano took up the fight in the courageous, energetic, positive manner in which he did, we *all* became Colts fans. *His* fight inspires me in *my* fight. Love having him for a teammate.

— **Stuart Scott,** ESPN anchor

Never in my thirty years covering the NFL have I seen the outpouring of feeling for one person as I did when Chuck Pagano was diagnosed with leukemia. Amazing thing is, so few people knew the man when it happened. Now, thankfully, you'll get to know Chuck Pagano and the fight he fought, and you'll be enriched because of his story.

— **Peter King,**
senior writer for *Sports Illustrated*

This would be a great read if it was just a thrill-packed, firsthand account of one the most dramatic football seasons of the past decade. It would be a great read if it was just an intimate, honest look at what it feels like to be locked inside a hospital room, literally fighting for your life. But this book manages, amazingly, to be both. You'll marvel at Chuck's grace and wit as he describes how he, his family, his doctors, and his team managed to beat both cancer and much of the NFL in one fell swoop. People have often asked me what it was like to be on the sidelines for many of the Colts' magic moments during the 2012 season. I typically reply, "You just had to be there." Now ... you can.

— **Rachel Nichols,** TNT sideline reporter
and host of CNN's *Unguarded with Rachel Nichols*

With *Sidelined*, my former coach, Chuck Pagano, moves the spirit like a great offense moving the chains. Coach is openly honest and relatable as he shares his battle with cancer and his craft of coaching in the NFL. *Sidelined* provides an introspective and unique avenue to get a front-row seat to faith, family, and football. Impactful!

— **Akbar Gbaja-Biamila,** former NFL defensive lineman,
current NFL Network analyst,
and cohost of *America Ninja Warrior*

Sidelined speaks to everyone looking to move through life with a positive, enthusiastic, and determined attitude. Coach Pagano tells his story of determination and victory and what it takes to be a true leader by demonstrating unmatched courage and dignity.

— **Bill Rancic,** entrepreneur

Chuck Pagano preaches family, and now he takes you inside his family in his touching story. Filled with inspirational tales and motivational messages, like CHUCKSTRONG, *Sidelined* is some kind of strong book.

— **Adam Schefter,** ESPN NFL Insider

Chuck's commitment and dedication to his family and his team during his battle with cancer is a true testament to his courage to rise above in times of uncertainty. He showed all of us that victory is achieved well beyond the fields of football.

— **John Fox,** head coach of the Denver Broncos

The CHUCKSTRONG movement that emerged less than a year after Chuck Pagano was named head coach of the Indianapolis Colts is indicative of the positive impact he has on others. Having played in the NFL myself, I can appreciate the strong bond between players and their coach. Chuck is a perfect example of a coach who cares for his team and brings out the best in others.

— **Mark Schlereth,** 12-year NFL offensive lineman,
two-time Pro Bowl selection, and ESPN analyst

Some people you work with, and some people you play with. Some people you are supposed to be with for a certain period of your life. Chuck is one of these for me. He is the total package. Chuck stands at all times for integrity and loyalty. I watched him go through extreme adversity, and he never once changed. I love this man and am honored to call him a friend. It is time for his testimony to be told. You will forever be changed.

— **Ray Lewis,** ten-time All-Pro linebacker,
MVP of Super Bowl XXXV, and ESPN analyst

Chuck is both a leader and great teammate at the same time. He lifts those around him to higher levels, and the world got to see that as he courageously battled leukemia. We can all learn from the way Chuck lives his life and leads his team.

— **John Harbaugh,** head coach of the Baltimore Ravens

It's been said a team will take on the personality of its coach. I've never seen a better example of a coach displaying mental and physical toughness, resiliency, optimism, and true grit through adversity than Chuck Pagano has shown to his Indianapolis Colts. His team has responded tremendously.

— **Steve Mariucci,** former NFL head coach
and current NFL Network analyst

Chuck Pagano epitomizes the best we all hope to learn from sports the day we sign up as kids. In a sport where the goal is to be tougher than the guy across from you, Chuck Pagano showed he was the toughest guy in any locker room in this league. Cancer definitely picked the wrong coach to pick a fight with. He's one of the rare guys in the league who left me feeling motivated every day I thought of him.

— **Jay Glazer,** senior writer for FoxSports.com
and NFL Insider for *NFL on Fox*

Coaches are too often measured by wins and losses. The coaches who truly make an impact are those who do far more than just lead their teams to victories. They are concerned more about the person than the player. They inspire, motivate, and challenge their players to be the best they can be — on and off the field. Chuck Pagano is certainly that coach. His greatest victory is the positive impact he has made in the lives of his players. In *Sidelined*, Chuck shares his powerful story of not only battling cancer but beating it as well. Chuck is an inspiration and a true example of being a great coach and an even better person.

— **Mark Brunell,** 19-year NFL quarterback,
three-time Pro Bowl selection, and ESPN analyst

Throughout my many years of playing in the NFL and during my time at ESPN, I've had the privilege of hearing some of the most amazing stories in sports. Chuck Pagano's journey of overcoming is one of the greatest out there. His sheer tenacity and drive are inspiring. This is a must-read.

— **Ron Jaworski,** 16-year NFL quarterback
and current ESPN analyst

Few men, if any, have inspired others within the NFL in recent years in the way Coach Pagano did. His 2012 Indianapolis Colts not only changed that franchise, but galvanized the entire league and those around it. We all became CHUCKSTRONG to one degree or another, and those postgame moments in the locker room when Coach Pagano spoke of his "circumstances" and his relentless will to coach again and see his daughters get married will always stand out to me as one of the priceless, signature moments of that entire season. Bruce Tollner's humanity, grace, compassion for others, and knowledge of the game make him uniquely qualified to help tell this story.

— **Jason La Canfora,** CBS Sports NFL Insider

I'm not sure I have ever been around someone who has such a contagious combination of fight and kindness. Chuck Pagano shares priceless lessons on how family, love, trust, and loyalty are critical components for facing life's greatest challenges. As a mother, wife, daughter, and former athlete, I found that *Sidelined* touched every part of who I am. Chuck gives us hope that cancer will be cured and we can win, inspiring us to put hope into action.

— **Heather Cox,** ESPN/ABC sports broadcaster

In his own words, Chuck Pagano reveals to readers his personal odyssey into and through the fight of his life. It was a story that not only dominated the NFL landscape but captivated the sports world as well. Only now do we learn the true details of the fight from Pagano's perspective. With unflinching candor and humility, Pagano inspires with his reliance on the three tenets of his life — faith, family, and football.

— **Sam Farmer,** *Los Angeles Times* NFL columnist

Chuck Pagano has always been a strong influence in my life (and in the lives of others too) as a father figure, a family man, and, most importantly, a teacher. When he was diagnosed with leukemia and then won his battle, it proved the strength and faith I knew he always had. He has always pointed me in the direction of helping the next person in any way possible. That's what makes "ChuckStrong"!

— **Ed Reed,** NFL eight-time All-Pro safety,
eleven seasons with the Baltimore Ravens

Chuck Pagano's story of recovery from leukemia is one that captured the nation in more ways than anyone could have imagined. His spirit and family values are to be admired. He's a true role model for fathers everywhere.

— **Adam Caplan,** ESPN NFL Insider,
SiriusXM Radio host, and member of the
Pro Football Writers of America (PFWA)

I couldn't put this book down. Between the lines of Coach Pagano's stirring account of his struggle to overcome leukemia during the Colts' remarkable 2012 season is a humble yet compelling message that extends far beyond football and into the faith and perseverance it takes to win in life.

— **Admiral James A. "Sandy" Winnefeld Jr.,** U.S. Navy

I'll never forget the day we announced Chuck's hire, and he addressed the full Colts staff in our pavilion. With almost no time for preparation, he went into full "coach mode" and, within a few minutes, had every person in the room, men and women alike, ready to strap on the pads and go kick butt for Chuck Pagano. But what took place when I visited him in the hospital reflects his true character more than anything. The first thing he wanted to know was how my family and I were doing. The man was in the fight of his life, and he refused to elevate his illness over his genuine caring for others. Astonishing and truly inspiring stuff!

— **Daniel C. Emerson,** vice president
and general counsel of the Indianapolis Colts

As a young graduate assistant at the University of Southern California, Chuck had a mind-set of, "I can do it; I will make it in the coaching profession." This story is a great example of what faith and a positive attitude can accomplish.

— **Ted Tollner,** veteran NFL
and college head coach

I followed Coach Pagano's story from the day it was announced he was battling cancer. But, his story took on a whole new meaning for me once I was able to sit down and interview him. Coach Pagano is a fighter — on and off the field. Following our interview, I kept repeating the same thing: *It's impossible not to play hard when you are coached by a man like that.* He truly inspires everyone he touches to fight as hard as he did.

— **Erin Andrews,** sports broadcaster,
journalist, and host on *Fox College Football*

Chuck Pagano's story is an inspiration to anyone looking for personal direction or a higher calling for themselves. As a son, brother, father, husband, leader, and coach, Chuck has a unique way of inspiring and bringing out the best in those around him. This is a story of inspiration and perseverance that will galvanize your spirit and warm your soul.

— **Terry Heffner,** Boise State University
wide receiver, 1986 – 1990

Chuck Pagano is one of the most passionate and courageous people I know. While battling cancer, he encouraged and supported those around him. And he inspired me like little else I have experienced. He reminded me it is the people in our lives who matter the most. Read *Sidelined!* You won't be the same afterward.

— **Pete Ward,** chief operating officer of the Indianapolis Colts

Having a small hand in the winning was rewarding; having a small hand in the healing is priceless.

— **Bruce Arians,** head coach of the Arizona Cardinals

SIDELINED

Overcoming Odds through
Unity, Passion, and Perseverance

CHUCK PAGANO
with Bruce A. Tollner

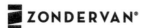

ZONDERVAN

Sidelined
Copyright © 2014 by Chuck Pagano

This title is also available as a Zondervan ebook.
Visit www.zondervan.com/ebooks.

Requests for information should be addressed to:
Zondervan, 3900 *Sparks Dr. SE, Grand Rapids, Michigan* 49546

ISBN 978-0-310-34106-2 (ebook)

Library of Congress Cataloging-in-Publication Data

Pagano, Chuck, 1960-
    Sidelined : overcoming odds through unity, passion, and perseverance /
Chuck Pagano.
        pages cm.
    ISBN 978-0-310-34103-1
        1. Pagano, Chuck, 1960- 2. Football coaches—United States—Biography. 3.
Leukemia—Patients—United States—Biography. 4. Indianapolis Colts (Football
team) I. Title.
GV939.P32A3 2014
796.332092—dc23   2014013121

Cover design: Curt Diepenhorst
Cover photography: SMI / Corbis®
Photo insert: Unless otherwise noted, all photos courtesy of the Indianapolis Colts
Photo insert background: Mario7 / Shutterstock
Interior design: Sarah Johnson

First printing May 2014 / Printed in the United States of America

My condition was being diagnosed with leukemia.
My position was fighting cancer
so that I would be around
for a long time for my wife and children.
My hope is that together
we can someday find a cure for all types of cancer.
Nobody should have to lose a loved one — especially a child —
to the bully called cancer.
To all the doctors, researchers, scientists,
caregivers, nurses,
and the millions of people
who so generously give to the fight against cancer,
I thank you.
This book is dedicated to you.

CONTENTS

FOREWORD BY TONY DUNGY

In July 2012, Jim Irsay, the owner of the Indianapolis Colts, invited me to Anderson, Indiana, to watch the team's first training camp practice under its new coach, Chuck Pagano. I was excited to go, not only to see some of my former players and staff, but also to get my first look at their new quarterback, Andrew Luck. But the highlight of my day was getting to spend some time alone with Coach Pagano in his office before practice. We had known each other and competed against each other over the years, but we had never had the opportunity to sit down for an extended conversation.

We talked about a lot of things that day, and I was amazed to find out just how much we had in common. Both of us had been longtime assistant coaches in the NFL before becoming head coaches. We both learned our craft on the defensive side of the ball and had worked for legendary, Super Bowl – winning coaches early in our careers. I learned under Chuck Noll with the Steelers, while Chuck had worked for Jimmy Johnson at the University of Miami. We both had tremendously supportive wives, strong women of faith, who encouraged us during every stage of our careers. Chuck's wife, Tina, sounded so much like my wife, Lauren, in the way she nurtured the children and worked hard at keeping the family together during the grind of so many long seasons.

As we talked, I also found out we shared a lot of the same beliefs about football and life. We both felt that you win in the National Football League by having good people who are united in a common cause. Yes, you have to have talented players, and you have to do things in a fundamentally sound way. And it takes preparation, hard work, and attention to detail to succeed. But in the end, having a team that functions like a family — a close-knit, loyal group that will not let each other down — those are the teams that win championships. But we also both believe that winning those championships wasn't the most important job of a coach. We talked about how the real joy in coaching comes from building relationships. Relationships with players, coaches, staff, and families that you can never replace.

As I went out to watch practice that day, it struck me as ironic that Chuck would be instilling those philosophies into the Colts' team exactly ten years after I started coaching with them. Jim Irsay hired me in 2002, after the team missed the playoffs, because he wanted his head coach to build relationships and develop a team that stuck together through thick and thin. The team bought into that philosophy and had a run of success that resulted in nine straight playoff seasons and two Super Bowl appearances. Now, a decade later, Coach Pagano was charged with reenergizing the team.

We did have an awful lot in common. But as I left practice that day, so impressed with what I had seen in the attitude of the team, I couldn't have known that in two months Chuck and I would have one more thing in common — a relationship with Dr. Larry Cripe, one of the country's foremost oncologists. In the summer of 2004, he began treating my dad, who had been suddenly diagnosed with leukemia. That summer, all the ideals I had talked about with our team for two years — about relationships and family being more important than winning games — got hammered home in a very personal way. Many of the players had gotten to know my dad, and we all learned firsthand the truth of those words. And now, unknown to any of us, God was about to show the 2012 team the same type of lesson.

Sidelined will show you what a close-knit family looks like. You'll see how the Pagano family, and the Colts family, dealt with adversity and didn't let it take them down, but instead used it to make them stronger and more unified. You'll be impressed with the inner strength and determination of Chuck and Tina. But I know that's not what they'll want you to come away with after reading this book. They will want you to see what God can do with a family, and a team, who have faith in God and a love for each other that can overcome even the toughest of circumstances.

FAITH, FAMILY, AND FOOTBALL

Like many coaches, I am a man who doesn't like to lose — or, at the very least, to not go down without a fight. It's not just my competitive spirit, although growing up in a football family, I'm sure that's part of it. I've always believed that perseverance, preparation, and determination — what we call "grit" on our Colts team — are not only essential but also contagious.

Growing up, I couldn't wait for fall to arrive so I could suit up for football. The start of the school year and a chill in the air always signaled a return to the gridiron. Now in my early fifties, I still get excited for a new season to begin, and I've been fortunate to enjoy that thrill as both a player and a coach.

One of the reasons I love football is that it's a team sport. Each man has to know his role, do his job, and give all he's got. Every player has to feel he's part of something bigger than anyone could achieve on their own. That's what winning is all about. The whole is always greater than the sum of its parts in any team sport, especially in football.

I've always viewed our teams as family. In order for team camaraderie to be real, there has to be trust. In order for there to be trust, you have to be committed to relationships. And lasting relationships require respect, dedication, and sacrifice.

Currently, I'm privileged to serve as the head coach for one of the greatest professional sports organizations in existence, the Indianapolis Colts. Coming from someone with only a couple seasons as head coach under his belt, this statement may sound like an exaggeration. But sometimes it takes going through adversity and overcoming it together for an organization — and its team members — to grow as a family. As I've always believed, circumstances don't make us who we are; they *reveal* who we are.

U

In 2011, the Indianapolis Colts struggled to a 2 – 14 record — worst in the National Football League. Another man who doesn't like to lose, team owner Jim Irsay, did not shy away from making some difficult decisions. In January 2012, Mr. Irsay chose not to renew the contracts of his president, general manager, and head coach. He wanted a new approach, a fresh start.

Like most Colts fans, he knew there was a winning tradition to maintain. From 2000 through 2010, the Colts won more regular season games (115) and had a higher winning percentage (.719) than any other NFL team. Winning remained deeply ingrained in the organization's culture. Under the leadership of Mr. Irsay, the Colts earned two trips to the Super Bowl, bringing home the championship trophy for the first time in three decades by winning Super Bowl XLI at the end of the 2006 season. So now, a 2 – 14 losing season was unacceptable. To get things back to normal, which to Mr. Irsay meant a winning season with a shot at a Super Bowl victory, everything became subject to change.

In January 2012, I was the defensive coordinator for the Baltimore Ravens. We had enjoyed a successful year of great football, culminating in the AFC Championship game against the New England Patriots, a game we came very close to winning. Once our season was over, however, I received a call from Ryan Grigson, the Colts' new general manager, asking if

I would fly to Indianapolis to interview for the available head coaching position.

After a long career of coaching football, I finally had a shot at my dream — becoming a head coach in the National Football League. My conversation with Mr. Irsay and Ryan Grigson went as well as it could have. Our conversation was candid, and I think we all knew we had found a rare opportunity for a unique partnership. Needless to say, it was the opportunity of a lifetime.

U

I knew the job would be challenging. Big decisions and more changes loomed on the horizon. Change is never easy, and while everyone in the organization welcomed me warmly, I sensed a "wait and see" approach to my leadership. I didn't blame them. They knew I had risen through the ranks as a defensive secondary coach before becoming defensive coordinator in Baltimore. They knew I had ties to coaches like Butch Davis and John Harbaugh. But any new leader tends to be a wild card until he proves himself.

After I was introduced as the Colts' new head coach in January 2012, I joined Mr. Irsay and Ryan Grigson in assessing the current players, the needs of our team, and our strategy for the upcoming draft in April. The biggest question revolved around the status of quarterback Peyton Manning. Once the anchor of a potent Colts offense, Manning had suffered a severe neck injury that forced him to sit out the entire 2011 season.

As the Colts' franchise player who led the team to all those wins beginning before the millennium, he had more than proven himself. But now we were at a crossroads. With Manning sidelined, simply put, the team was unable to put enough points on the scoreboard to win. After missing the entire season, would he be able to return from such a debilitating injury, repeat his past performance, and sustain his success over several more seasons? No one knew.

In March 2012, Mr. Irsay made the decision to release Manning.

Obviously, this wasn't an easy decision to make, and initially our fans expressed both sadness and anger, but releasing Manning allowed us to use our No. 1 pick in the NFL Draft to select Andrew Luck, Stanford's standout quarterback, who was the Heisman Trophy runner-up in both 2010 and 2011. If Andrew was as good as we believed he was, he would become our franchise quarterback, a pillar around which we could build our offense.

U

From the first day when I arrived in Indianapolis, Mr. Irsay, Ryan, and I talked about how we wanted to build something special — not just another powerful football team, but one that resembled a family unit. Certainly our focus would be on winning football games — that's the objective of the business we're in. However, to succeed in the NFL, winning goes beyond the X's and O's and putting great athletes on the field. Every franchise has great athletes. That's a given.

To have a championship team, it takes camaraderie and a strong bond that the players and coaches have for each other. To achieve this we created a family environment, one in which everyone cares for his teammates. We strived to build a brotherhood of men and an environment where everyone was aligned, always moving in the same direction. Yes, we knew there would be speed bumps along the way that would slow us down but wouldn't stop us. When everyone has the same beliefs, you unite. You galvanize.

I had no idea how quickly our new family's bonds would be tested. Three games into the regular season in the fall of 2012, I went to see a doctor, who ordered some tests to be run. The results, as you may know, were not good. I was diagnosed with acute promyelocytic leukemia — APL for short. A cancer of the blood cells.

Suddenly, I was sidelined.

U

When the Colts' organization learned of my diagnosis, they reacted like a true family and gave their unconditional support. I happened to be the one who became ill, but had it been any other member of our family, I know the reaction would have been the same. What happened next, in my life and in the life of the team, exceeded everyone's expectations, and with the help of my good friend, Bruce Tollner, I'd like to share our amazing journey.

Much of what I experienced confirmed what I believe and how I try to live my life. While some of the special moments can't be put into words, I've discovered that much of what I learned about battling cancer and winning football games applies to whatever you're facing in life. As you'll see in the following pages, I believe we can all beat the odds. My hope is that what I share will inspire and motivate you in the same way that faith, family, and football continue to inspire and motivate me.

CHAPTER 1

LET'S HUNT

Arriving in Indy

Dedication is not what others expect of
you; it is what you can give to others.

—**Anonymous**

T he storm was over.

When training camp opened in late July 2012 in Anderson, Indiana, the oppressive heat from a summer drought scorched the Midwest, turning our practice facility into an oven. Talk about trial by fire for a rookie coach. But then two weeks into camp, a massive rainstorm blew in, powerful enough that we had to cancel our afternoon practice. Thunder echoed across the campus of Anderson University, the site of our preseason camp, as lightning crackled against angry, dark skies. High winds drove much-needed rain into the area and cooler conditions for the rest of camp.

Some of the sports media called the storm a symbol of the "winds of change" taking place within the Colts' organization. I liked the comparison because we definitely wanted to lay the foundation for a new era within our program, a season of change.

By the final day of camp in August, the hot sun returned, an appropriate omen for the battles that loomed before us. A new season was about to begin, and it was clear that no one would be satisfied with a repeat of the previous year's performance, particularly our team's owner, Jim Irsay.

Mr. Irsay knows football like the back of his hand. He was twelve years old when his father, Robert Irsay, a Chicago businessman, purchased the Baltimore Colts in 1971. As a young boy, he cleaned locker rooms, picked up towels, ran errands, and learned the business from the ground up. He received a degree in broadcast journalism in 1982 from

Southern Methodist University, where he played linebacker for the Mustangs. An ankle injury ended his playing career, but he never left the game.

When he finished college, Mr. Irsay joined the Colts' organization in 1982. Two years later, at age twenty-five, he was named vice president and general manager just weeks before the Colts moved from Baltimore to Indianapolis. He then became the team's chief operating officer after his father suffered a stroke in 1995. When his dad passed away in 1997, Mr. Irsay gained 100 percent control of the franchise. At age thirty-seven, he became the youngest team owner in the NFL.

After seeing his beloved Colts go 2 – 14 in 2011, Mr. Irsay took dramatic risks to implement a new season of winning ways. He made many personnel changes, one of which opened the way for me to be hired as head coach. In addition to betting on me to lead his team, Mr. Irsay also chose another rookie, thirty-nine-year-old Ryan Grigson, to be the team's general manager.

During his college days, Grigson played tight end and offensive tackle at Purdue. In the 1995 NFL draft, the 6-foot-5 college standout was drafted in the sixth round by the Cincinnati Bengals. He later played for the Toronto Argonauts of the Canadian Football League and retired in 1997 due to a back injury. Ryan took a job as a pro scout for the Saskatchewan Roughriders and then worked as an assistant coach for McPherson (Kansas) College in 1998. After holding various scouting jobs in professional football, the Philadelphia Eagles hired him to be a scout in 2004, and in 2010 he was named director of player personnel, where he remained until he joined the Colts a few weeks before I arrived.

U

I'm well aware of the gamble Mr. Irsay took in hiring me as well. I am not what you'd call an overnight success story. In 1984, I earned my first job as a graduate assistant at the University of Southern California. Ted Tollner, my friend Bruce's father, was the Trojans' head coach and a great man to break me in. Coach Tollner inspired me to consider coaching as a career, saying, "Chuck, you keep working as hard as you can and pouring all you've got into the game of football. You've got what it takes to lead a team someday."

But I had a lot to learn. So I worked hard to break down game films, prepare scouting reports, coach the scout team, and generally assist the position coaches. As one of the four graduate assistants, I was also the team's gofer. I'd take the laundry out and pick up lunches. On Halloween I'd get pumpkins, and on Christmas I'd get Christmas trees. It was not a very glamorous job, and it involved a lot of grunt work. This is how you break into the business on the coaching side. So coaching became the way I sustained my love for football.

Before coming to Indianapolis, I had been coaching for twenty-eight years. During that time my family and I moved twelve times. After spending two years at USC, I served another year as a graduate assistant under the legendary Jimmy Johnson at the University of Miami. The following two years, I coached linebackers at Boise State — and that's where I met my wife, Tina, who was born and raised in Idaho. In 1989, I coached defensive backs at East Carolina and then spent the next two years at the University of Nevada, Las Vegas (UNLV). In 1992, I went back to East Carolina for three years to coach defensive backs and linebackers, and from there back to the University of Miami, where I coached defensive backs and coordinated special teams for six years under head coach Butch Davis.

My first National Football League job was with the Cleveland Browns after Butch Davis was named head coach. He hired me to coach the defensive backs, which I did from 2001 to 2004. Next, I spent two years with the Oakland Raiders coaching defensive backs. When Butch Davis was named head coach of the University of North Carolina in 2007, he chose me to be the Tar Heels' defensive coordinator for one year, and then in 2008, I was hired by the Baltimore Ravens as a defensive backs coach. In 2011, I was promoted to be the Ravens' defensive coordinator — a job I carried out during a season in which we came within seconds and a few feet of a goalpost of earning a trip to the Super Bowl.

The Ravens were 12 – 4 during the 2011 season and earned a bye going into the playoffs. Playing New England in the AFC championship game, we were down 23 – 20 late in the fourth quarter. Our quarterback, Joe Flacco, stepped back to pass and hit Lee Evans in the end zone — for the touchdown that would have sent us to the Super Bowl. The ball zipped straight into Lee's hands, but he couldn't secure the catch before a Patriots' defensive back knocked the ball away. Pass incomplete.

But we still had a chance to tie the game. Our kicker, Billy Cundiff, had made this kick 99 out of 100 times — an "automatic" boot through the uprights. But not that day. The kick sailed wide to the left. Instead of the game going into overtime, the Ravens' season ended. We would not be going to the Super Bowl as we'd all hoped and expected. We were all devastated.

U

The day after our loss, head coach John Harbaugh summoned me to his office. "Chuck, the Colts' general manager Ryan Grigson called me and wants to talk to you. They're doing a head coach search, and they want you to go to Indianapolis for an interview."

I was totally surprised. I didn't even know they were looking for a head coach! I still had my blinders on. Our Ravens squad had been focused on one thing and one thing only — to win the Vince Lombardi Trophy. I was struck by the irony. If our receiver had held on to that ball in the end zone, or if we had made that field goal and gone on to win in overtime, I would be focused on preparing our defense for the Super Bowl and the Colts would likely have not called.

However, other circumstances prevailed, and I trusted God that they were for the best. I called Ryan, who said Mr. Irsay wanted to talk to me. Ryan had similar thoughts to my own. Right off the bat he said, "I know the loss to the Patriots stings for you and the Ravens. If Billy Cundiff had made that field goal and the Ravens had won, you'd be on your way to Indianapolis to play in the Super Bowl and this telephone conversation would not be happening."

Prior to my interview, Mr. Irsay had asked Ryan to do a background check on me. He made phone calls to several players and coaches who had worked with me over the years. In 2010, when Ryan was with the Philadelphia Eagles, they were interested in hiring me as their defensive coordinator, and by the time of the interview he had accumulated a sizable file on me. Mr. Irsay asked Ryan to sit in on the job interview, along with Pete Ward, chief operating officer and a thirty-year veteran with the organization, and Dan Emerson, a vice president and the Colts' general counsel.

I had little time to think through the interview and went to Indianapolis cold, not as prepared as I like to be. Opportunity rarely knocks under perfect conditions, though, and I was grateful for the meeting. We met in a boardroom, where Mr. Irsay and Ryan immediately made me feel comfortable. Mr. Irsay talked about faith, family, and football. He explained his vision for the future. He was very passionate about his team and very direct about what he expected in the near future.

Mr. Irsay also talked a lot about his family members and asked questions about mine. I was thoroughly impressed with how important family was to him. Similarly, Ryan Grigson and his wife, Cynthia, have five children, and it was obvious that his first priority was also his family. Pete Ward and Dan Emerson were clearly strong family men as well. We all shared the same values and clearly hit it off at that first meeting.

I did have one prepared question to ask: "The Colts are a great passing team. I'm a defensive coach. Why aren't you talking to a coach with an offensive background?"

"We know we'll have a great quarterback and a strong offense," Ryan answered. "We want a great defense to go with it. We want balance, and you've done a great job with the Ravens. Baltimore has such a strong defensive culture."

Mr. Irsay also said they liked my reputation for being able to connect with my players. "You have consistently developed a mutual respect with them over the course of your career," he said. "We're looking for a leader of men."

Near the end of our conversation, Ryan scribbled a note on his legal pad and put it in front of Pete Ward, the Colts' COO. Pete read the note and nodded. We finished the meeting, and

Mr. Irsay called the next morning to offer me the job as head coach of the Colts. We talked about the details, and I asked him if I could have a little time. "I need to sit down with my wife and talk to her about this," I said. Mr. Irsay told me to take my time and call back after I talked with Tina.

∪

After a couple of hours, I called Mr. Irsay back. When he answered the phone, all I said was, "Let's hunt." This was an expression used a lot during my time in Baltimore. It was our way of letting each other know it was time to go to work, time to eat! This phrase signaled it was time to get in the game and be as focused as possible. When I said, "Let's hunt" to Mr. Irsay, he knew I meant I was accepting the job, that I was ready to go to work.

Mr. Irsay told me I was exactly what the team needed to move forward. "Ryan and I had many discussions about what we wanted in our head coach. At one meeting Ryan asked me, 'Is there someone out there who can charge up the side of that hill with sword in hand and lead his men into battle? Someone who can take that hill and emerge victoriously — no matter the odds?' His question made an instant imprint in my mind of the kind of leader we needed. Someone who had that kind of charisma, leadership, and passion to fearlessly lead a charge, no matter the circumstances. We believe you fit that bill, Chuck. From the minute we sat down and talked to you, and from all the feedback we've gotten about you, we believe you have these unique and special traits we want in a leader. Dan and Pete were impressed by your passion — we all were."

I was speechless, humbled and honored by what he was saying.

After a short pause, Mr. Irsay continued. "We were looking for someone who truly cares about the players and wants the best for them. That's why we believe you are our man. I connected very quickly with you and knew I wanted you to be our next head coach. Your love for this great game was evident from the start, and your personality is one I know our players and fan base will identify with. Beyond your passion and skill as a coach, you're also a relatable guy!"

When Mr. Irsay said this to me, I knew I was at the right place. I also knew they had big expectations for me, and I would do whatever it took to not let them down. Later, after I arrived in Indianapolis, Ryan showed me what he had written on that note he handed Pete during my job interview. It read, "Players will run through a brick wall for this guy."

Ʊ

Having spent twenty-eight years in the football business following my college graduation, I was once asked if I had always wanted to be a head coach. This is a question I always ask when I interview an assistant coach. I want to hire coaches who are great teachers, love what they do, and strive to be the very best at their craft. Coaches who aren't afraid to fail, who are driven to one day lead their own teams. People who are dedicated to the pursuit of excellence in all they do, individuals committed to working together as part of a team to create something bigger than themselves. So in a sense, yes, I've always wanted to be a head coach, determined to work hard and keep reaching for the next level.

With these qualifications in mind, one of the first calls I made after taking the job was to my old friend and colleague Bruce Arians, the man I wanted as my offensive coordinator.

Following a track that was similar to that of my own career, Bruce had spent his entire life in football, dating back to when he was a top scholastic quarterback at York Catholic High School in York, Pennsylvania. From 1972 to 1974 he was the starting quarterback for the Virginia Tech Hokies and stayed on as a graduate assistant for two years until he got an assistant coaching job at Mississippi State University, where he worked with running backs and wide receivers.

From there, Bruce coached running backs under the legendary Paul "Bear" Bryant at the University of Alabama in 1981 – 82. Then from 1983 to 1988, he was the head coach at Temple University, where he compiled a 21 – 45 record. In 1989, he worked for two years as a running backs coach for the Kansas City Chiefs and then took a job as the offensive coordinator from 1993 to 1995 at Mississippi State. He spent a year as a tight ends coach with the New Orleans Saints, another year at Alabama as an offensive coordinator, and then two years as a quarterbacks coach with the Colts. During this period between 1998 and 2000, he was Peyton Manning's first quarterbacks coach in the NFL. From 2001 to 2003, Arians was a quarterbacks coach with the Browns while I was in Cleveland, and that's where we became good friends.

Bruce joined the Pittsburgh Steelers in 2004 and worked as the wide receivers coach, and then for four years he was the Steelers' offensive coordinator. Having seen how he coached Ben Roethlisberger to so much success, I knew Bruce was the man we needed to help develop the young talent on this team and run our offense.

As we would discover several months later, Bruce's contribution to me and to the team would become more than either of us could've imagined.

U

I first began to notice something wasn't right toward the end of training camp. Feeling fatigued and exhausted, I assumed it was from the fifteen-hour days of meetings and two-a-day practice sessions. My excitement and adrenaline kept me going, but when I saw the unexplainable bruises on my torso, arms, and legs, I wondered what was going on. *Maybe I'm not eating enough of the right foods or my body's running low on iron or some other vitamin or mineral,* I thought. Like most coaches would do, I just kept plugging away and working to get better. I've yet to meet a player who wants to leave the game, and I wasn't about to do so either.

Overall, camp had gone really well, and I was grateful for the opportunity to be more hands-on. The hardest part of my first few months as head coach had been administrative. In addition to hiring Bruce, there were other coaching staff positions to fill, tasks to delegate, and information to learn about the organizational side of the team.

I also invested a lot of time in getting to know the players and was happy to sign defensive lineman Cory Redding, defensive tackle Brandon McKinney, and safety Tom Zbikowski. All three came from the Ravens' defensive unit, and I was excited about continuing to work with such talented defensive players. I knew they would be a huge asset in building our Colts defense, and transitioning from a 4 – 3 alignment to the 3 – 4 scheme that had been so effective for many years in Baltimore.

On the offensive side of the ball, I also enjoyed getting reacquainted with Reggie Wayne, the Colts' superstar receiver whom I'd known back in his University of Miami days in the late 1990s. I had been the secondary and special teams coach there and recognized the amazing talent and professional-career potential in Reggie even then. While he was excited about my being his coach again, Reggie reminded me that I had changed in the dozen years since we had worked together, which I hoped was for the better. "You're still loud, direct, and demanding like you were back then," he told me with a grin, "but you're also more invested in your players. I love the way you still get a kick out of the game, the way guys improve a little each day."

Our new quarterback, Andrew Luck, was proving to be both the talented athlete and team leader we hoped he would be. He was impressive throughout camp, completing 319 of 447 passes with 28 touchdowns and nine interceptions in team drills there in Anderson. While I was well aware of his stats, I just liked seeing the ball spinning out of his hand and making its way into the hands of our receivers.

U

As training camp drew to a close, I looked forward to returning home and getting ready for our first preseason game quickly approaching. I was eager to see Tina and the latest changes she had made to our new home. While coaching certainly takes a toll on anyone, I'm convinced its greatest impact may be on coaches' wives and their children. Tina bore the brunt of handling all the details of moving from our home in Baltimore, having now become a veteran of a dozen such transitions.

I also wanted to get my wife's input on why I hadn't been feeling well. She knew as well as I did the toll of long days and late nights in professional football, and she always did a great job making sure I was taking care of myself, at least as much as possible under the circumstances. Besides, the bruises and fatigue were probably nothing. Considering the circumstances, who *wouldn't* be exhausted? I was in a new job — we all were — and pushing ourselves harder than ever.

So I attributed my fatigue to the long hours I was putting in, coupled with little sleep. I had been going to football training camps practically all of my life, and feeling exhausted at the end of the day was the norm. But something seemed different this time. I continued to find more bruises on my body — deep, dark purple bruises. They were slow to heal, and I didn't have the slightest idea where they had come from.

I wasn't getting hit on the playing field, and I didn't recall bumping into anything. Maybe I had been more physical on the field at training camp than I'd realized. *I've been bruised many times*, I thought to myself, *so I can't worry about some black-and-blue marks. They'll go away. I just need a few good nights of sleep.*

But after making the hour-long drive from Anderson back to Indy, I could never find the time to slow down. The preseason was about to start, and the regular season immediately after that. I was determined that our team would get off to a great start. So I just kept going. When I wasn't on the practice field, I was attending meetings, studying film, and coaching the players. We were all working nonstop, seven days a week. Like any all-consuming career, with coaching it's not like you can just call in sick.

In hindsight, I was like every other hardheaded, driven individual who ignores the signals our bodies try to give us.

No way was I going to let some bruises slow me down. I'd just keep going and not pay any attention to them.

But my bruises didn't go away. They signaled the arrival of something much more serious. Something that could not be ignored.

CHAPTER 2

WINDS OF CHANGE

Beginning the 2012 Season

Success is not final; failure is not fatal: it
is the courage to continue that counts.

—Winston Churchill

Any time you build something new, you have to begin from the ground up. With training camp under our belts, it was now time to test the foundation we had been laying for the past eight months. With the support of Mr. Irsay and Ryan, we overhauled many of our team's systems and strategies. For the first time in over a decade, the Colts would be implementing new systems for both our offensive and defensive units. We rearranged the locker room and tried to make it clear that it was a new era, a fresh start. In the weight training room, we had the words "Trust," "Loyalty," "Respect" — the core pillars for our team — painted in big letters beneath the Colts horseshoe.

The winds of change clearly swept over our entire team as well. Only twelve players remained from the 2009 Super Bowl team. We brought out ninety men to training camp, and more than sixty were new to the organization. More than a third of them had never played in a regular season NFL game before. The franchise quarterback, Peyton Manning, had been released and had chosen to sign with the Denver Broncos. The man we hoped would become the same kind of successful team leader, Andrew Luck, was smart, talented, and dedicated — but still untested.

During training camp, Andrew had demonstrated the kind of poised performance we hoped to see from our No. 1 draft pick. He was a natural leader on and off the field, with a hunger to win and a contagious determination to do whatever it takes to win as a team. And he began his NFL career with the same kind of stellar performance as his legendary predecessor, Peyton Manning.

The rookie quarterback opened our first preseason game at home against the St. Louis Rams. He dumped the ball off to Donald Brown, who ran untouched 63 yards for the team's first score. Andrew ran down the field with the entire offense to congratulate Brown. What a great way to start! He went on to play an incredible game, connecting with Austin Collie in the end zone on our third possession, followed by a steady, calculated 80-yard drive for another score after a Rams field goal. We couldn't have asked for a better way to begin. Ranked dead last in the Associated Press Pro32 poll, we clearly surprised everyone, especially our exuberant fans.

This game reinforced what we had been preaching for the past seven months. We had more talent and determination than anyone gave us credit for. Eager to show everyone our brand of Colts football, we wanted to make it clear we were going to decide the outcome by how we played and executed. And it would not be determined by the so-called "experts" and analysts.

U

Some fans believe preseason games don't matter, that they're just a few warm-up exercises before the real season starts each September. But they're more than just a dress rehearsal for the actual games looming ahead. I remember a reporter asking me how many exhibition games would be the right amount for our team, and I answered, "Ten!" I was only half kidding, because we really do need all the playing time together we can get. Preseason games aren't just about going through the motions for when it counts; they're about practicing the skills, putting in the work, and building confidence and trust in one another.

Our second exhibition game didn't go as smoothly as our first. We visited Heinz Field in Pittsburgh to take on the Steelers, which is always a challenge for any team — whether in a preseason or regular season game. Even though we lost the game by two points, we saw many signs of growth and improvement. One of the most significant was our quarterback's ability to bounce back after making the rookie mistake of throwing a short pass intended for receiver Reggie Wayne right into the hands of defender Ike Taylor, who ran it back for a pick-six, an interception returned for a touchdown by the opposing team's defense.

But Andrew has one of the rare gifts that make quarterbacks great — amnesia. While aware of his mistake, he wasn't paralyzed by it or afraid to risk playing at peak performance out of fear it would happen again. He had a veteran's sense of calm maturity. He knew, like we all knew and like anyone who follows football knows, interceptions happen. You hope they're few and far between, but mistakes are part of the game. More importantly, Andrew knew that learning from your mistakes and not letting them get in your head are what elevates champions above the rest.

U

For all practical matters, by the time we finished the second exhibition game, I felt like the season had started. Like a train picking up speed as it leaves the station, football season accelerates until everything else feels like it's a blur. I was excited, focused, and passionate about our team. We had good men on board who clearly shared the same vision, work ethic, and determination to win that Mr. Irsay, Ryan, the other coaches, and I all shared. We had been fortunate to bring in some defensive players I already knew, mostly from my time in Baltimore. These veteran players already knew what the rookies were discovering — we play to win and never, ever give up, no matter how big the score or how little time remains on the clock.

The pace continued to leave me feeling tired and drained of energy. I assumed it was just the grind — long days, short nights, meetings, practices, poor eating habits, and not enough exercise. But the bruises continued to appear on my body. Tina had noticed them by this time, but I had downplayed them as "no big deal, probably caused by getting bumped on the field during practices." They continued to nag at me in the back of my mind, however, and I promised Tina that if they didn't go away in another couple of weeks, I'd ask a team doctor to take a look at them.

In the meantime, only a couple of weeks remained to prepare for our season opener against the Chicago Bears. While we continued to improve in our final two exhibition games, it felt like two steps forward and one step back — but at least we were making progress. We lost our third preseason game against the Redskins in Washington, but continued to learn a lot from our mistakes.

Lots of media hype and fan interest had surrounded the game because of the matchup between the two superstar quarterback draft picks going head to head, our Andrew Luck against their Robert Griffin III. Both rookies played like seasoned leaders on the field, and I continued to be impressed by Andrew's ability to rebound from his mistakes. He remained nimble, quick on his feet, and incredibly accurate in his ability to execute plays and find an open man downfield. He was exceeding expectations and making it clear the Colts were not going to be the doormat that everyone expected us to be.

We concluded the 2012 preseason with a win at home against the Cincinnati Bengals. Overall, I was pleased with the progress we had made in the past month. The real test, though, would be the matchup against the Chicago Bears at Soldier Field. Although we finished the preseason at 2 – 2, the performance of our quarterback and the improvements emerging out of our new offensive and defensive systems had raised everyone's hopes.

U

My first regular season game as an NFL head coach did not go according to plan. In fact, it was nothing short of a nightmare. Everything that could go wrong went incredibly wrong. Sacked three times and knocked to the ground repeatedly, our rookie quarterback threw for only one touchdown while suffering three interceptions — not all his fault — and one fumble. Our defensive backs were flagged for pass interference and holding multiple times. The momentum and synchronicity that had developed in our preseason seemed to evaporate during four agonizing quarters at Soldier Field.

That Sunday night and the following Monday were spent sifting through the wreckage and performing an autopsy on our numerous mistakes. It was probably the first time the team saw me really frustrated and upset. I told them, "We couldn't beat the local high school team with five turnovers! I don't care who you're playing, we must take care of the football, not commit foolish penalties, and not beat ourselves. You don't win games in the NFL; you lose them."

But what I loved about the team's response is that everyone took responsibility. Andrew Luck assumed more than his fair share of the blame. We all know how hard it is to win when you lose the turnover battle, especially if you end up minus four for the game. Obviously, we needed to improve in all areas in a short amount of time. But the attitude of our team and coaching staff after that initial loss was to go to work and get better. We were all determined to make amends for our first performance of the season. This was not the kind of football any of us expected to play. This was not Colts football. We all held ourselves to a higher standard.

Despite losing our first game with such a dismal performance, our guys responded with a gritty determination to learn and to improve. As painful as it was to watch the film, there was no other place I wanted to be. We all knew this team could win, and we were determined not to let one loss set the tone for our season. We had work to do, but the men were willing to do it.

You can tell a lot about a person's character by how they respond to defeat and disappointment. Some coaches rant and rave, curse and blame, and try to motivate their team into a better performance. But this has never been our style. We win as a team, and we lose as a team — period.

In hindsight, many positives came out of losing our first game. We got to see each other in the heat of actual play for the first time. We learned how we responded as individuals to disappointment, and more importantly, we grew in our resolve to improve as a team. The guys saw that while we all wanted to win, we wanted to do it as a team. Every single one of us would need to improve and contribute if we wanted the Indianapolis Colts to be a great team. No one man could carry the team, but every man working together could achieve greatness.

U

Our follow-up response in our home opener against the Minnesota Vikings proved we were serious about our commitment to winning as a team. Playing against a stout Vikings defense led by Pro Bowler Jared Allen and an offense anchored by premier running back Adrian Peterson, we had our work cut out for us. But we played solid football and clearly had improved by focusing on our fundamentals after the loss to the Bears. Our offense performed up to its potential, and we entered the fourth quarter up by two touchdowns.

However, with slightly more than 5 minutes left in the game, the Vikings made it clear they weren't giving up without a fight. They matched our two touchdowns and tied the game with less than a minute left to play. But Andrew and our team were not about to let this game slip through our fingers. After two 20-yard completions, he drew the Vikings' defense offside and then spiked the ball with 12 seconds remaining. Clutch kicker Adam Vinatieri booted the ball 53 yards through the uprights, and we had our first regular season win.

While we celebrated the victory, the following day I emphasized one of the keys to becoming a championship team. I told the guys you can't get too excited after any win or too down after any loss. You've got to stay the course if you want to keep getting better, week in and week out. Take each week as it comes, and don't become overconfident after a win.

Stick to the process, and never get too high or too low. One game at a time. Stay humble, and work each day to get better. The rest will take care of itself.

Besides, with our next game against the Jacksonville Jaguars quickly approaching, there was no time to dwell on last week's win. On paper, this game appeared to be one we should win. The Jags had lost both of their games to that point and were clearly experiencing some growing pains under their new regime. But they also had one of the league's most explosive running backs, Maurice Jones-Drew, who I refer to as a rolling ball of butcher knives. With his power and speed, MJD could decimate a defense and change the entire tone of any game. Heading into a game you're *supposed* to win always makes you nervous.

Ʊ

We had a right to be concerned. Maurice Jones-Drew had a great game, rushing for 177 yards. Despite having made progress with our defense, we couldn't contain him, but somehow he didn't seem to be the reason we lost the game. Even with the success he had running the football, we managed to keep it a close game. By the end of the fourth quarter, we were down 16 – 14 with only minutes to go. Our offense quickly moved the ball, covering 48 yards in five plays. With 56 seconds remaining, Vinatieri kicked a 37-yard field goal, and it looked like we were going to win by one, as we were up 17 – 16.

So we kicked off deep into the end zone, forcing a touchback. The Jags had to start their drive on the 20-yard line. With the clock at :56, everyone on our team was collectively holding their breath. You learn that anything can happen while there's still time on the clock, so nobody was celebrating yet. But it was within reach, and we could almost taste it. Until that one play.

Jacksonville quarterback Blaine Gabbert threw to Cecil Shorts III on a post pattern, and — *unbelievable, are you kidding me?* — it's an 80-yard touchdown! One play. That's why it's the NFL. On any given Sunday any professional team can beat another, no matter who has the better record, the most statistical talent, or greater depth at key positions.

But it wasn't over yet. We still had almost 40 seconds on the clock, and our offense seemed more determined than ever to make the most of them. Down 22 – 17, we were back in the game as Andrew completed six consecutive passes. On the final play of the game, however, he threw a 26-yard strike to Reggie in the end zone that Jags cornerback Aaron Ross broke up. In football, so much can happen to win or lose a game in only a matter of seconds.

We were now 1 – 2.

U

In the locker room after the game, our spirits were down. I made a few remarks but kept them short. Then Robert Mathis, a thirty-two-year-old linebacker and one of our team leaders, stepped forward and demonstrated why he's such a great leader. "There are no pity parties in football," he began. "Let's man up. We'll look at the tape, make the corrections, and move on."

I'll never forget that. It was like a scene from a movie, and a screenwriter couldn't have scripted a more powerful, motivational message. Robert's few, well-chosen words spoke to the hearts of his teammates and lifted our mood. Yes, we had work to do, but that's why we were there! The season had barely started. We simply had to learn from this game, make the necessary adjustments, and move on.

Despite the second wind Robert's words breathed into us, the next day I was especially tired, and my thoughts returned to a conversation I'd had with a team doctor the previous morning before our game. Since the bruises had not healed, I finally showed them to a doc on staff.

"How long have you had these?" he asked.

"You know, I can't answer that. I'm not exactly sure," I said, "but a fairly long time. I remember noticing them at the end of training camp."

"I want to draw some blood and do some labs," he said. "We'll do that on Tuesday morning."

I agreed, primarily because we were approaching our bye week and I didn't feel as rushed as usual. Had it not been a bye week, I probably wouldn't have gone ahead with it. But on Tuesday a nurse came to the complex to draw blood, and then that night, the team doctor called with the results.

"Chuck, some of your counts are off," he said. "I'm scheduling you for an appointment tomorrow."

"What do you mean when you say 'off'?" I asked.

He hesitated for a second. "Your platelet count is around 20,000, which accounts for the bruising. Your hemoglobin and white blood cells are also outside normal ranges."

At the time I had no idea what that platelet number meant, but hearing the concern in his voice got my attention.

"I made an appointment for you to see Dr. Larry Cripe at the Indiana University Simon Cancer Center. Be there tomorrow after morning practice."

"Tomorrow? Can't this wait? Who did you say I'll be seeing? What kind of doctor is he?" The alarm was finally starting to go off in my mind. This wasn't a little thing I could just ignore. I wouldn't be able to take some iron supplements and forget about the bruises. Something else was going on. Something much more serious.

"Dr. Cripe is a hematologist and oncologist, and he's the best in his field."

Taking a deep breath, I said, "You've got to be kidding me."

"I'm sorry, Coach," he said. "I wish I was."

CHAPTER 3

THE BYE WEEK

Or How I Became The Rock

Resilience is accepting your new reality, even
if it's less good than the one you had before.

—Elizabeth Edwards

I didn't tell Tina about my blood count.

I was sure it would turn out to be something minor, so I figured, *Why worry her about nothing?* Looking back, I confess there was an initial sense of denial on my part. I thought, *Hey, I'm a football coach — I'm in decent shape. What could possibly be wrong?* Something in me clearly wanted to hang on to that youthful notion that we're all invincible. Only I was reaching a point where I knew that wasn't true.

So the next morning, a Wednesday, I tried to act like it was just any other workday. But when I arrived at our training facility, I was forced to recognize that everything was about to change. When it was time for my appointment, Dr. Robertson from our team medical staff walked into my office and said to me, "Where's your wife? Is she here? She's gotta take you."

I just looked at him for a moment, wondering if he knew something I didn't. Then I said, "I haven't told my wife. I don't want to scare her. She doesn't need to worry about this, so I'll just drive myself down there."

"No, you can't," he said firmly. "Call your wife and get her over here. She has to take you." His tone clearly indicated this was simply the way it had to be. I'm just as stubborn as the next guy, if not more so, but I knew better than to argue this time.

"Hey," I said after Tina picked up. She was just finishing up the women's Bible study she holds at our house every Wednesday during the season. "I've got an appointment with a doctor at the IU medical center. I was told not to drive myself, so I wonder if you can pick me up and take me there."

Silence. Then Tina calmly said, "I'm on my way."

One thing I love about my wife is the way she rolls with the punches. After more than two decades of marriage, we've learned how to understand each other beyond the words we say. She knew something was up.

U

On the ride to the hospital, I told Tina about everything leading up to this appointment, well, with the exception of my blood counts.

In her usual calm way, she casually asked, "What kind of doctor is Dr. Cripe?"

"A hematologist," I said, trying to sound just as matter-of-fact. "You know, a blood specialist."

"Why a hematologist?" she asked.

"Better safe than sorry," I replied just a little too quickly.

My wife wasn't fooled. She knew we were venturing into uncharted waters. A few minutes later, still on our way to the Indiana University Simon Cancer Center, Tina said something to me I will never forget: "Chuck, look at all we've gone through over the years. All the moves we made. How hard you've worked your whole life. You finally get the opportunity of a lifetime and then something bad happens. I just can't believe God brought us here for something bad to happen. I just can't accept that."

Tina and I are very positive people, largely because we share a strong faith in the Lord. We don't wear our beliefs on our sleeve or try to force them on others. We just try to place our trust in God and let our actions reflect our beliefs.

After meeting Dr. Cripe, however, I began to wonder. We got acquainted, but he quickly cut to the chase.

"Chuck, I saw the results of your blood work, and we're

going to draw blood again and also do a bone marrow biopsy. But I want you to know beforehand that I'm 99 percent sure you have acute promyelocytic leukemia — APL for short."

Tina and I looked at each other, and neither of us said a word. We didn't know what APL was, but the word *leukemia* jumped out at us.

"What are you saying?" I asked.

"Let's see the results after we do the biopsy," he said in a calm voice.

After the blood tests had been completed, Tina and I sat in the reception area waiting for the results. It was all so unreal. This couldn't be happening to us. I had a new job I absolutely loved; things had really come together for us; and I was more content than I'd ever been.

U

"Yes, that's what you have."

We were back in Dr. Cripe's office. He went on to describe how leukemia originates in the body's bone marrow, where normally we churn out billions of cells that mature into red and white blood cells. Leukemia arises when the production of white blood cells goes awry. The rogue cancerous cells proliferate, crowding out the normal blood cells and taking over.

"What we have to do," Dr. Cripe explained, "is give you chemotherapy treatments that concentrate on knocking out those cancerous cells so the normal cells take over once again."

We listened carefully, too stunned to say anything. "Those bruises you have," he continued, "are a result of blood clotting or bleeding problems, and they're consistent with acute leukemia."

Dr. Cripe took a brief pause and continued. "APL is very

curable. Here's what we have to do. You're going to be in the hospital, probably for about a month, and we're going to start you on chemo ASAP. I'm sending you downstairs immediately, where we're going to put in a PICC line for you to receive chemo through. It's a small line we'll place in your upper arm."

Unbelievable. It was all totally surreal. We had a few seconds to sit there and digest what just happened. All I could think about was Tina and our children. *What would happen if ...?* Dr. Cripe sounded very knowledgeable and credible, but still. *Leukemia.* I couldn't imagine how I would tell our daughters.

"Tina, you'll need to go home and bring back some things for Chuck to get settled into his room," Dr. Cripe said, continuing to move at lightning speed with my entire life. "You don't have to bring everything today."

For some reason, that comment sent me over the top and momentarily broke the spell. "Wait a minute," I exclaimed. "Just hold on a minute, Dr. Cripe. You're going too fast. I can't just drop everything! I have too many things on my plate."

He started to speak and paused, and then he looked me in the eye very calmly and respectfully said, "Chuck, this isn't something that can wait. You're welcome to a second opinion, but I promise that you'll get the exact same results. You're going to be in this hospital for about a month or so." He looked over at Tina, letting me absorb the impact of his words. "Everything else must be put on hold."

Visibly shaken, Tina said, "We will do whatever is necessary to get Chuck well again."

"We'll get the admissions process started immediately," the doctor said, "and we'll start doing a series of tests so we can begin the chemotherapy."

"Wait a minute," I said in a way that must have sounded like I was pleading. "Can we just go home together and get some things and come back?"

"Chuck, you can't leave," Dr. Cripe said firmly. "It's too dangerous. Your counts are outside the normal range, and your immune system is shot." He made it clear I was putting my life at risk if I didn't stay in the hospital.

I thought through the chain of events that would domino from this news. "We've got a lot of phone calls to make," I said. "We have to let our three daughters know what's happening. There are my parents, my family, and Tina's family. And the team — I have to let the team know about it ..."

And to think — I was going to drive myself to this appointment. Everything can change in a matter of moments. *Everything.*

U

I made the calls to our daughters. My wife made the calls to my parents in Boulder, Colorado, and to her family in Idaho. Thank God for Tina. I'm not sure I could have gotten through all those calls by myself. I'm not sure how she did it.

The upside of my diagnosis was starting to sink in. Dr. Cripe said APL is a very curable cancer when it is diagnosed in time, and in my case, this meant the odds of survival were in my favor. However, he also said that to beat the disease, I would receive heavy doses of chemotherapy that would kill the bad cells and in the process also wreak havoc with my immune system. As a result, I would be very sick for several weeks before I'd begin to feel better.

It never entered my mind that I would not survive my cancer. I had my wife, my kids, and my grandkids to think about, and I had to be there for them. My thinking was, *I will beat this*. Tina knew my favorite mantra going into tough games: "We can! We will! We must! By any means necessary — we have no choice — *we will win*." Suddenly, its meaning on the football field paled in comparison to what was at stake. I had no choice but to beat this thing. I had to — for my family.

The rest of that day felt like a blur. After leaving Dr. Cripe's office, I was wheeled downstairs, where they put a bracelet on my wrist and put me in a room. Then they immediately brought in all the necessary machines that would soon start dripping Idarubicin through the PICC line they had put in my arm, along with steroids and other antibiotics to fight off infection. My first chemotherapy treatment was about to begin.

I had time, and I needed to make one more call. Ryan answered on the first ring and said, "Hey, where are you? I've been looking all over the place! I've got some ideas I want to run by you." Our offices have connecting doors, so we see each other about fifty times a day. When we want to talk, we just walk into each other's office.

"Well," I said, "I'm down at the Simon Cancer Center."

"What are you doing over there?"

"Uh, are you sitting down?" I asked.

"Yes, I'm sitting down," Ryan said. "What's going on, Chuck? You better not be joking with me!"

As I began to tell him about the cancer diagnosis, he clearly knew I wasn't joking. He remained quiet for a long few seconds and then said, "You've got to be kidding. Please tell me you're not serious."

"I wouldn't joke with you about something like this."

I could tell by his voice that what I had told him floored him.

There was another silence, and I remained quiet so Ryan could grasp what I had said. We had become very close friends over the past nine months, and I knew he cared about me and my family.

When Ryan and I came to Indianapolis, we both lived here for several months without our families. Ryan and I stayed in condos while our wives and children were in the East, selling our houses, packing our things, and getting ready to relocate. Both he and I came in to the office in the early hours of the morning and stayed until late at night. We had enjoyed many late dinners together, and we continually texted and talked after we both got home. It was difficult to tell him about leukemia because I knew he'd take it hard. Ryan was a kid when he lost his father to cancer, so I knew how he'd react to the news.

"I'm about to start my chemotherapy, so I'm not going to be able to call Mr. Irsay and some of the others," I said. "Ryan, I'm counting on you to let the team know what's happened. Tell them that I don't know when I'll be back, and it might not be until the end of the season."

"You just get better," Ryan said, "and we'll figure out what to do in your absence. The most important thing right now is for you not to worry about the team. Your health is the number one priority."

He paused and I could hear a crack in his voice. Then he continued. "Coach, I've got you covered. I'll call Mr. Irsay, and we will make all the adjustments that have to be made."

Ʊ

Ryan and I cut through the emotion and briefly discussed who should step in for me. We both agreed Bruce Arians, our new offensive coordinator, would be the right man for the job.

Ryan promised to relay our thoughts about Bruce being my replacement to Mr. Irsay. Although Mr. Irsay always sought our opinions prior to making a decision of this magnitude, he was the team owner, and ultimately it would be his call.

Owning an NFL team is big business, but it's also a people business. There is nobody in the league I respect more than our team owner because his top priority is building relationships with his people. He truly cares about everyone, and this caring attitude permeates throughout the organization. He cares about his people, and they feel the same way about him. I knew he meant it when he later told me, "Chuck, I'd trade places with you if I could."

It was no surprise that Mr. Irsay and his family were the first people to visit me when I was admitted to the hospital. He assured me that my job was secure and said, "If there's anything I can do for you and Tina, just name it, and it's done."

"We could use your prayers," I said.

"You're in them," he replied, "and I'll keep on praying. But whatever I can do to make you more comfortable, I want to do that." He paused and then added, "Your children live out of state. How about if I bring them in on my jet?" Sure enough, the following week, on my birthday, October 2, he sent his jet to pick up our daughter Tori and bring her to Indianapolis for a visit. Our two other daughters weren't able to make it, or he would have flown them in too.

U

"I'm looking for The Rock?" said a nurse with an amused expression. I gave her a funny look in return. "Or do you prefer Mr. Johnson?" she continued. "Or just Duane?" She marched in and began to check my vitals. "See," she said, gently twisting my ID bracelet so I could read it. Sure enough, typed there was JOHNSON, DUANE — AKA "THE ROCK."

I laughed for the first time that day. "What in the world? Who came up with The Rock?" I asked.

"Your wife," said the nurse, smiling at us. Apparently, while I had been getting my PICC line put in, another nurse had stopped in my room and asked Tina what alias I wanted to use. Because no one except our immediate family, Mr. Irsay, Ryan, and the Colts' top executives knew about my diagnosis and hospital admission, we wanted to keep it quiet until all the players and other coaches were notified. If I'd been admitted under my own name, with Twitter and all the social media sources, the news would have leaked out, and the team would've found out the wrong way. Mr. Irsay wanted to make a personal announcement at a special team meeting he'd called.

"The Rock?" I asked Tina, still smiling. "Really?"

"You know I'm a fan!" she teased. "And I knew it would make you laugh."

U

That same day, on September 26, I was given a room in the intensive care unit at the Indiana University Simon Cancer Center and received my first chemotherapy treatment. With heavy doses of chemicals in my bloodstream with a mission to destroy the cancer cells, I was told my immune system would be compromised. To prevent exposure to viruses and germs, I would remain in the unit for an unspecified period of time. In order to create a germ-free environment, flowers and fruit baskets sent by players, coaches, team executives, and fans were not allowed in my room.

Dr. Cripe told me I'd be very sick once the chemotherapy

kicked in. And he was right. After a few days, I began to feel the effects of the chemotherapy and couldn't believe how it sapped every ounce of energy. Early on, I had fluid in my lungs and needed oxygen. I wasn't afraid really; it just felt like my life — my *real* life, where I was married to Tina, the father of three beautiful daughters, and the head coach of the Indianapolis Colts — had been placed on hold.

From a mental standpoint, I was able to deal with all of it because I have been hardened from having been an athlete and a football coach. But the physical part? It was hard dealing with the daily grind of feeling like someone had beat the — well, you know what I mean. The vicious cycle reminded me of the movie *Groundhog Day*. They would give me medicine to handle a side effect of chemo. Then they'd give me another medicine to deal with the side effects from that medicine, and later, yet another for *those* side effects — and the cycle continued.

Soon I completely lost my appetite. My taste buds were gone, and I had no desire for food. I heard that some people on chemo get a lot of sores in their mouth and even their esophagus so they chew on ice for relief. Thank God that didn't happen to me. It didn't hurt for me to chew or swallow so much; I simply didn't have the desire or energy to eat.

From that first night in the hospital, Tina slept in my room on a small couch that could seat two people. It could be turned into a bed, and the medical staff brought in sheets and a blanket for Tina so she could make it up every night. Her rest was interrupted the same as mine. Neither of us could get a good night's sleep because the nurses came into the room every couple of hours to check on me and get vitals. Not that we would have been able to sleep much anyway, with so much weighing on our minds.

U

Now, I've never been one to hide my emotions. I cry at most weddings, and sometimes when I watch a sad movie — well, my eyes have been known to water just a little. Tina and my daughters know I love an emotional story, that my passion for life runs deep and I'm not afraid to show it. I just never had to face a challenge like this one in my own story before.

After the dizzying, rocket-speed appointment with Dr. Cripe, Tina and I had finally had an emotional meltdown that first day in the hospital room. We just looked at each other, and Tina said, "I'm so sorry this happened to you. I'm just so sorry."

That did it. The love she conveyed at that moment just wrecked me. We both started crying. After a few minutes, I wiped my eyes and I said, "Okay, now that we got *that* out of our system."

Tina wiped away her own tears and said, "We just need to do whatever we have to do to get you home." After that afternoon, I never saw Tina cry again during my illness. Just recently, she told me she was able to control herself in my presence because she knew it would break my heart to see her so sad. She said, "I reserved my tears for when I was driving home to take a shower or do the laundry."

Her support was unbelievable. I knew our love was strong, but you never appreciate someone's love the way you do when it's tested by this kind of trial. "I want to know everything they're doing," she told me. "Absolutely everything you're going through. I have to be here so I know." She felt confident about the care I was getting, but she wanted to see firsthand what was going on.

As a result of her dedication, whenever a doctor or a nurse

came in the room to give me medicine, Tina would ask, "What are you doing?" She wanted to know everything and didn't care what they might think. "Why *that* medicine? What does it do? What are its side effects?"

Prior to my illness, Tina didn't know a thing about cancer. She had no reason to; she had never been around anyone who had cancer. But now, she was like a student in medical school — always asking questions, researching, and reading. Eventually, listening to her talk with Dr. Cripe and other medical staff sounded like a foreign language to me.

A few days into my treatment, Tina entered my room and could tell I had reached a new low. "How are you feeling?" she asked, squeezing my hand.

I just shook my head at first and then managed to whisper, "I've got nothing today. Nothing." I didn't want to tell her, but I had started to wonder how I was going to endure the remaining weeks of chemo. I knew I had to do it, but I couldn't imagine how. This battle was without a doubt the hardest thing I had ever faced.

And it was just beginning.

CHAPTER 4

ORANGE GLOVES

The Team's Response to My Leukemia

The most successful people are those
who are good at plan B.

—James Yorke

In less than a week, I was exhausted from the chemotherapy. Sometimes I was able to get up and take a sponge bath; other times it took all I had to go to the bathroom or brush my teeth. Some of the simple things I had taken for granted became a chore. The oral chemo known as ATRA gave me migraines. Then the docs ordered pain meds, so I'm doped up and can't go to the restroom so they start giving me something else to help me go to the bathroom. There were aches and joint pain. And the night sweats, the fevers. I'd wake up in the middle of the night absolutely soaked. Then I'd get up, have the chills, put on dry clothes, and have to do it all over again a couple hours later.

Tina started a routine for us each morning. Every day we'd have devotional time together, reading or listening to books like *Jesus Calling* and *Our Daily Bread*. We prayed a few short sentences or just sat quietly and prayed without saying any words. While the alias on my ID bracelet may have read, "The Rock," we both believed that Christ is the solid Rock who would see us through this.

After our devotional and prayer time together, I usually had a visit from Dr. Cripe or one of his medical team. I remember after the first few days of my treatment he said to me, "I know you're an important person, but I don't know anything about football."

"No, I am not," I replied. "I'm like everyone else. I'm just a patient. I'm just somebody here to beat cancer."

"Just know," he said, "that our number one goal is to get you better and take care of you."

71

I couldn't have asked for a better doctor — not only one who was an expert oncologist but one who took the time to get to know me and understand a little bit about my life. Right from the beginning, Dr. Cripe told us what the game plan was and what we had to do. "Our goal is to cure you," he stressed, "not just treat you."

"What are my chances?" I asked. "What's the survival rate — statistically?"

Dr. Cripe just looked at me thoughtfully and then said, "Our goal is to cure you. Period."

Eventually, I found out that according to the American Cancer Society, early treatment for APL, which may include chemotherapy and drugs like all-trans retinoic acid (ATRA), as well as transfusions of platelets or other blood products, brings remission in 80 to 90 percent of patients. I knew, all things considered, these were favorable odds. But there was still that other 10 to 20 percent.

Right away Dr. Cripe requested that a whiteboard be posted on my bathroom door with a calendar to chart my progress. Starting on Thursday, September 27, 2012, I was able to check my white cell count and my hemoglobin and platelet values. I paid close attention to those numbers, praying they would move in the right direction.

U

The same day I received my first chemotherapy treatment, Mr. Irsay summoned Bruce Arians to his office, and when the meeting came to an end, our new offensive coordinator became the Indianapolis Colts' interim head coach. At age sixty, Bruce was at a point in his career where he had stopped worrying about becoming a head coach in the NFL.

Following the meeting, a blast of emails, texts, and follow-up phone calls went out to everyone in the Colts' organization. Mr. Irsay called a mandatory team meeting for the following Monday morning, unusual because we were on our bye week, which meant players had extra time off to spend with their families. Everyone knew something was up.

Visiting me shortly after that meeting, Cory Redding, our 6-foot-4, 315-pound defensive end, described that meeting. Cory's a special guy, and we had become good friends back in Baltimore when I was coaching the Ravens' defensive unit. Cory's contract had expired at the end of the Ravens' season, and after I joined the Colts, I asked him to join us in Indianapolis. In addition to being an incredibly strong, intense player, Cory possessed excellent leadership qualities, the very kind of traits we needed to help build our Colts squad, to support the type of culture and environment we wanted in our organization.

Cory has always been generous in his support for me, and now would be no exception. I'd read interviews in which he'd tell reporters, "Chuck is almost like a player in the D coordinator's position. The guy has so much fun with us. He treats you like more than a player. It's like we're his sons. He wants us to do well. He keeps it fresh. He knows everybody's strengths and puts them in a position to make plays."

Cory went on to comment about why he came to the Colts: "A lot of people talk about family, but they don't walk the walk. Chuck really is into serving others. At training camp, he emphasized serving each other, and he showed us what that looks like firsthand. He told us, 'Sacrifice. Give up everything you got for the man next to you, your brother, and know he will do the same for you.' Chuck really brought this message home in everything we did. It was never about 'this is my team' and 'you do as I tell you to do,' or 'do this or do that.' That's not who Chuck is.

"His style reminds me of when I was a kid. Everyone in the family had a role, and the parents were the ones in charge. We could have fun with Mom and Dad, but they're still the authority, the ones I had to answer to. This is how Chuck treats the guys on his team. We know he's the head coach and wears the big hat. At the same time, he gets down on the level of the rookie, the second-year, and third-year guy — as well as the ten-year guy — and he has fun with all of us. Chuck lets it be known that even though he's your head coach, he will always treat you respectfully, man to man. The guys respond positively to that. When Chuck asks you how your family is doing, he's not just making conversation. He truly cares about your family. You can't fake this kind of stuff. Chuck simply brings a family atmosphere into the building."

U

Here's how Cory described the special team meeting that took place on that Monday morning:

"After our bye week Wednesday morning practice wrapped up, by noon everyone — the players and coaches — took off to enjoy a long weekend. Some of the guys were going home, with plans to be back in town by Sunday night. My wife, Priscilla, and I were headed out of town, and on Friday she had sent several text messages to Tina. 'How's your bye week going?' my wife texted, and then when she didn't hear back, she sent another message: 'I'm just checking on you.' Tina didn't respond, and Priscilla was concerned. It wasn't like Tina, who'd always got right back to Priscilla. They were friends from our time together in Baltimore and stayed in touch pretty regularly.

"Over the weekend I received a phone call and was told an emergency team meeting was scheduled for Monday morning at eight. When I asked what it was about, I was told I'd find out at the meeting. This wasn't the usual way people in the Colts' organization talked to one another so I knew something was up. I checked in with some of the guys on the team, and they'd received the same call — but no one got any details either.

"So Monday morning, I walked in a few minutes early and started looking for Coach, but he wasn't there, which was also weird. Chuck's usually standing in the front of the room ten minutes before any meeting starts. I figured he must be talking to Ryan or Mr. Irsay, so I took a seat and waited.

"A few minutes later, Mr. Irsay entered and went to the front of the room, followed by Ryan. Then we saw that all the coaching and training staff people were in the team meeting room as well. Next all of the other executives entered the room. Still no Chuck. I knew something was terribly wrong. This wasn't just any kind of typical team meeting.

"After all the players and staff had gathered, Mr. Irsay nodded to let everyone know he was going to speak, and there was a hush in the room so quiet you could hear a pin drop. Mr. Irsay said, 'Coach has been feeling some fatigue over the last few weeks, and he's noticed some bruising on his body. At first he thought the bruises could have been from contact on the field, or coaching, or playing with his grandkids. After he showed them to Tina, she made him promise to get them checked out. Coach saw one of our team doctors, who ran some tests and referred Coach to be evaluated by a specialist. We now know that Coach has leukemia.'

"The room grew completely still, as Mr. Irsay continued. 'Obviously, this is a difficult blow for him and his family. It's unlikely he will be able to coach again this season. With any battle against cancer, there are peaks and valleys. And once he gets better, there's more chemotherapy to go through. We all know the demands of this league. It's one of the most demanding jobs anyone can have. While Coach Pagano receives treatment and recovers, Bruce Arians is going to be our interim head coach. He is Chuck's selection and certainly has my blessing, along with Ryan's.'

"Mr. Irsay paused briefly, his emotions beginning to overcome him, and added, 'I feel in every fiber of my body, and I know Chuck feels the same way, that he can beat this thing.'

"I was stunned. Coach was healthy last week, and now he's fighting for his life. It was hard for me to accept. Chuck and Tina had become like family to Priscilla and me. Sitting there in the awful silence of Mr. Irsay's announcement, I said a prayer for Chuck, for Tina, for their entire family. This was all so unreal. Then I had a thought that gave me comfort. Back in my early football days, I'd learned that when you face adversity, you really only have two choices: you either fight or you fold. There was not a doubt in my mind about which one Chuck Pagano would do. He's a fighter through and through."

U

After Mr. Irsay's announcement at the team meeting, he asked Bruce Arians to say a few words. Bruce made it clear to the team that I was the Colts' head coach and he was just filling in until I came back. He announced he had switched on the light in my office, and it would remain on, 24/7, until I was healthy and on the sideline coaching the team again. When I later heard about my office light being left on, I loved the powerful display of support and the visual reminder of my presence being with the team even though I wasn't in the building.

Coach Arians concluded by challenging the players: "We can't control whether Chuck can make it back before the December 30 regular season finale, but there's another option we can control. We can *extend* the season until he's with us again on the field!" He was talking about making the playoffs, a lofty goal for a team that had gone 2 – 14 the previous year and was currently 1 – 2. But we had been conditioning our players to think big for eight months.

Over and over again, we'd been telling them, "Stick to the process. It's sixty minutes, all you got. One play at a time. Don't judge. No matter what happens, good or bad, move on, next play. If you're up or you're down, whatever — just play one play at a time." As simple as it may sound, I firmly believe this is what commitment to excellence and dedication to our team are all about. This is what we do, week after week. We stick to the process. Win or lose, this is our routine. Stay the course.

From day one, Bruce and I stayed in touch by means of phone calls, emails, and texting on a daily basis. He said to me, "You coach your ass off from the couch, and we'll handle the rest. Don't worry. The job's gonna get done."

He visited as much as possible. Our conversations were about the Colts, but they were also personal. "How's Tina?" Bruce would ask. "And how are the girls?" Bruce had survived prostate cancer a few years earlier, so he knew what I was going through, and we often talked about my treatments. As much as we talked about the Colts — and that was a lot — there was still a clear sense of what matters most. Football is not who we are; it's what we do. As players and coaches, it doesn't define us. Family does. Faith does. You're defined by *how* you play the game, not by the game itself.

U

After the team meeting, the Colts held a press conference to explain to the media all that was going on. I asked Dr. Cripe to make a statement, and he agreed. He informed the many reporters, "I met with Coach Pagano last Wednesday when he was evaluated for bruising, and that evaluation demonstrated changes that were consistent with acute leukemia. He was hospitalized Wednesday night, and we began treatment at that time. I'm here today because the coach has asked me to be here. He wants to deal with this challenge in a very forthright fashion. Before I explain the treatment and diagnosis in general terms, I would like to emphasize a few things.

"First of all, the goal of the treatment I'm about to describe is to cure the disease. A cure means Coach Pagano returns to a fully functional life — the life he's worked so hard to enjoy. And he's looking forward to leading the Colts to some Super Bowls. However, the process is long and complicated, and we're just starting right now. So for the next several weeks, the process will be day by day. We'll be vigilant, and we'll do everything we can to help him reach full recovery."

Dr. Cripe explained that my cancer was of the bone marrow tissue, the source of my bruising. He told reporters I was in the induction phase, which has a goal of complete remission and normal blood counts. Dr. Cripe said this phase typically lasts four to six weeks and that once it was completed and I was stable enough, I'd be able to return home and continue treatment on an outpatient basis.

Dr. Cripe concluded by saying, "I'm not a big NFL fan, but I know the life of a coach is pretty arduous. I don't know when Coach Pagano will feel well enough to resume full responsibilities, but I know he's anxious to return in any capacity he can. However, his health is obviously the priority. Chemotherapy and recovery will take several months. I don't think Coach Pagano will be doing any serious coaching any time soon."

Our general manager Ryan Grigson then spoke briefly and said the fighting spirit I bring to football will be applied to my medical condition. "Chuck's a fighter," he said. "The best medicine for him is for the team to continue to fight for four quarters."

U

Bruce Arians also made a brief statement at the press conference, reiterating what he had said to the team about setting a goal to extend the season to the playoffs so I could be there on the sideline with the team. By saying this, Bruce made it clear to the press and our fans that our goal was to be a strong team in 2012. This was consistent with every message I had made since being named head coach. From the time I came to town, we never said that the 2012 season would be a rebuilding year. We only talked about winning.

In fact, we never used the "R" word ("rebuilding") in the building. Not in a meeting, not out in public. And never to the media. We were not there to rebuild; we were there to reload. We wanted to win every game. And if we didn't win this week, then we were going to go back to work, make corrections, get better, and prepare to win next week's game. This was our mission. Right from the get-go we had a vision. Nobody thought that, given a 2 – 14 record the previous year, the Colts could have a winning season in 2012. We believed differently. We all believed.

Prior to the regular season, we had a media breakfast where a reporter asked me, "Coach, with all the changes, with all the turnover of people, with all the circumstances, with the condition your team is in, are you going to lower your expectations?"

"To answer your question," I replied, "I want to invite you to come with me to our next team meeting. You can personally tell our players they should lower their expectations." He declined my invitation. He didn't want to face guys like Cory Redding, Robert Mathis, Reggie Wayne, Dwight Freeney, and Antoine Bethea and say that. I talked to this reporter about our vision, our ultimate goal, and the only reason we sign up. "Playing and coaching aren't for everybody," I said. "It's tough. It's hard. It's hard to win football games. It's a grind. But the reason we do it is to hoist the Lombardi. We want to dance under the confetti. We want to get in the tournament, get hot, and win it all. That's our goal."

U

Later I learned how other players reacted when they heard about my illness, especially the guys I knew really well. For example, there was wide receiver Reggie Wayne. Like my relationship with Cory, my relationship with Reggie had been a close one for years, long before I came to Indianapolis, so he took the news especially hard. Reggie told me what went through his mind at the team meeting when Mr. Irsay made the announcement:

"I knew from the moment the owner walked into the room and you weren't there, Chuck, that something was wrong. When Mr. Irsay told us about your diagnosis, instant tears came to my eyes. My first reaction was, 'Why Chuck?' I've been around leukemia. It took three people I was close to. It just wore them down. It defeated them. So I know what it can do. I couldn't help thinking I'm 0 for 3 with leukemia.

"I'm thinking, 'Chuck always goes around with a big smile on his face. He enjoys life. He preaches all the right things. Why him?' It didn't make any sense. So I closed my eyes and put my head down. Everyone took the news so hard. That room was so quiet you could have heard a mouse piss on cotton! This news just sucked all the air out of the room. And I couldn't hold my emotions back. When the meeting was over, I bumped into Coach Arians, and we were both crying. We had a practice later that afternoon, and it was probably the worst practice I've ever had in my professional career. I was dropping balls, running the wrong routes. The news had affected me big-time."

Reggie and I met when I was coaching at the University of Miami during his college days, and we have been close ever since. Since I was a defensive coach and he was a wideout, I never actually coached him at Miami. But we just hit it off, and over time we developed a close relationship. Reggie describes our special bond by saying, "We're family. It's not a coach and player. I know his wife and kids. I know about his dog. We are not related by blood, but I look at him the same as family."

Reggie's play on the field speaks for itself. He is a tremendous athlete and a great football player — and one of the most competitive guys I've ever been around. But you know what? He's an even better person. He's a fine young man with high character. I'm a relationship guy, and I have always tried to build strong relationships in every job I've ever had. To my good fortune, Reggie is a part of my life.

Reggie was a first-round draft choice of the Colts in 2001, and in 2012, at age thirty-four, he was admired and respected throughout the league. The younger members of our team especially looked up to him. In early 2012 when I came to Indianapolis, Reggie was a free agent, so he didn't have to stay with the Colts. He was an All-Pro receiver, and several teams were eager to sign him. So when I got the job, one of the first calls I made was to Reggie.

He has since told me that when his phone rang, he could see on his caller ID that I was on the line. "I knew why you were calling, and I didn't want to answer the phone!" he laughed. "I wanted to throw the phone in the ocean because I knew how hard it would be to say no to you." After the Colts' horrific 2011 season, I understood why Reggie would want to sign on with a team that was a Super Bowl contender, and a lot of teams out there were interested in him. "Hey, Reg, I don't want to do this without you," I said. "I'm asking you to just take a leap of faith."

He could have easily joined a team with a proven quarterback. As one of the game's top receivers, Reggie would have been a great addition to a lot of offensive units in the league. He could have chosen from a handful of offers from already proven teams on the cusp of heading to the Super Bowl. But instead, he took a chance. And now suddenly, I wasn't going to be directly coaching him after all.

But Reggie never regretted his decision to stay with the Colts. When the announcement of my illness was made, he announced he would dedicate the rest of the season to me.

"When Coach Pagano first started talking about how the Colts could be playoff contenders," he told a reporter, "I didn't buy into it immediately. But once I got to training camp and saw the guys we had around, and saw the scheme, I felt like we had some good things in place. I'm a believer."

U

Determined to support me during the rest of the season, Reggie came up with an idea he wanted to implement in our next game after the bye, our October 7 game against the Green Bay Packers. He knew that the NFL regularly partners with the Susan G. Komen Foundation in the fight against breast cancer each October, which is Breast Cancer Awareness Month. You may recall noticing on the field the bright, fluorescent pink shoes, socks, towels, sweatbands, and other apparel each October to help raise awareness for the fight against breast cancer.

Aware of the attention the pink accessories attracted, Reggie did a little research and discovered that orange was the color designated in the battle against leukemia. He knew the NFL maintains a very strict policy about what players are allowed to wear on the field, but in this case he didn't care. "I knew I might get fined for violating the NFL uniform code, but if they fined me, I would just have to pay it. Since I didn't want it to come across as disrespecting the team, though, I told Bruce Arians what I wanted to do. 'Do you have a problem with it?' I asked him. 'Hell, no!' he said, and then added, 'Wish I'd thought of it!' "

To support me and to raise awareness in the fight against leukemia, Reggie was inspired to wear bright orange gloves in Sunday's game against the Packers, knowing as a receiver, his hands would definitely get noticed by the crowd and the cameras. He asked our equipment guys if they could make some orange gloves for him, but they were unable to do so on such short notice. So they made calls to several teams that had orange as one of its team colors — the Miami Dolphins, the Cincinnati Bengals, and the Denver Broncos.

The Dolphins sent Reggie Wayne half a dozen pair of special gloves used by their receivers — all in bright orange. To make sure he was comfortable with them, Reg used them in practice the day before the Packers game. The last thing he wanted to do was drop balls coming his way because he wasn't used to the new gloves. He told me later he felt a lot of pressure going into that game, wanting to do his absolute best.

He was not the only one. The Indianapolis Colts were about to show the world how a family takes care of its own — by going out as a team and winning as a team. Reggie had no idea how much his orange gloves would come to mean to me.

CHAPTER 5

CHUCKSTRONG

Why Beating the Packers Was More Than Just a Win

To succeed you need to find something
to hold on to, something to motivate
you, something to inspire you.

—**Tony Dorsett**

From the time I arrived in Indy, we constantly talked about *trust, loyalty,* and *respect.* We became committed to these core values. Underneath the horseshoes you see in the weight room, these three words summarize how we play and why we play — trust, loyalty, respect. How we treat each other, how we conduct ourselves both on and off the field, how we go about our business on a daily basis.

They're not just for players and coaches. They apply to everyone in the entire organization, and everyone has to buy in. Everyone has to know that his or her job means something, and this applies to the people behind the scenes, not just those who are on the football field. We want *everyone* to know that no role is insignificant and that when we succeed, everyone contributes to our success and shares in celebrating that success. From the time Mr. Irsay, Ryan, and I first talked about what we wanted to achieve, we were determined to create a culture where guys couldn't wait to come to work. We wanted people who would be excited about getting up in the morning and being here.

We had long conversations about this kind of environment. None of us wanted the kind of place where people stand around a watercooler complaining about their jobs or disrespecting the organization and each other. When people are unhappy at work, they let their coworkers know about it, and their families as well. And simply put, a "misery loves company" attitude is contagious — and deadly. There's no quicker, easier way to divide a team than to ignore the mortar that holds the bricks together.

Trust. Loyalty. Respect.

We wanted a workplace where people are honest and forthright with each other. We wanted open communication to be practiced daily. We wanted every person in the building to be treated with the dignity that every human being deserves. Sure, we're tough guys, and we like to joke and trash-talk sometimes as part of our fun. But there has to be a limit to that kind of behavior, and we wanted everyone to respect each other more than anything else. A joke's only funny if we all share in it together at no person's expense. And when we make mistakes or do something wrong, we don't deny it. We want a place that if we are going to eat crow, we are going to eat it while it's hot!

This is what we wanted, but anybody can talk about it, put these words on paper, and paint them on a wall. Trust, loyalty, and respect have to be earned. You can't buy the value they carry. They're earned by walking the talk, not talking the talk. Every one of us has to do the right things — players, coaches, *everyone*, and you do these things day in, day out.

Talking about these things doesn't cut it. While open, regular communication is vital, you must live out the values, or you're not going to get a group to buy in. You won't have a team of people who can face adversity and have everyone working together to overcome it unless there's a true bond forged by a mutual commitment to shared values.

Prior to my battle against leukemia, I had no idea just how important those values would be to me and to our team. And I never expected to see them lived out in such amazing and bold ways. I never imagined being at the center of a movement called CHUCKSTRONG.

U

Reggie Wayne wasn't the only player committed to spreading the word about fighting leukemia and beating cancer in my honor. Pat McAfee, our punter, tweeted several messages to his followers about my condition and encouraged them to show support for me by joining the battle to fight cancer. He ended his tweet with #Chuckstrong. It caught on — in a big way.

By midweek, a few days before our upcoming Sunday home game against the Green Bay Packers, a CHUCKSTRONG campaign had started selling T-shirts, wristbands, and banners in the Colts' pro shop, with proceeds going to leukemia research. Inspired by Lance Armstrong's LIVESTRONG campaign, organizers of CHUCKSTRONG announced there would be huge CHUCKSTRONG banners with orange ribbons behind both goalposts.

The media jumped on the opportunity to expand the campaign and its impact. Various media personalities told fans to show their support by wearing something orange to Sunday's game. It could be a T-shirt, wristband, cap, tie — anything as long as it was orange. They told fans, "Think about Chuck and Tina in their hospital room, watching the game on television and seeing a sea of orange!" Tina and I were overwhelmed with emotion when we heard about this.

In addition to CHUCKSTRONG, the support we received from the people of Indiana was mind-boggling. I couldn't thank them personally — there were literally thousands of people who wanted to encourage us, so I thanked them in a letter I sent to the *Indianapolis Star*:

All the cards, gifts, emails, success stories, and prayers that
we have been showered with give us a tremendous amount of
peace and strength. We could not get through this without you.

Later that week I sent another message to the newspaper,
and I urged the sellout crowd to get into the game and help
inspire the team to upset the favored Green Bay Packers: "May
the 12th man be stronger than ever," I wrote. "You will make a
difference. Need to hear you from Room C231 at Simon Cancer Center. Let's hunt!"

In still another email I sent to the *Star*, I wrote, "All is
good," and about my treatment I wrote, "Best care in the world.
These people do so much for so many. Most selfless people I
know. Thanks to all at IUH [Indiana University Health Simon
Cancer Center]!!"

Meanwhile throughout the week I had been getting my
daily chemotherapy treatments, which continued to have side
effects that made me feel weak, nauseous, and exhausted. I was
also losing weight, and my hair was beginning to fall out. But I
tried my best to keep my focus on the team — first, because I
wanted to help the guys in any way I could, and second, I knew
being involved from my bedside would be a good distraction
from my illness. I figured that by being busy, the time would
go faster and I'd be able to get out of there and feel better again.

So I frequently sent text messages from my hospital bed to
the players and coaching staff. Often my texts to Bruce were
along the lines of, "Tell this guy this and that guy that." Bruce
diligently relayed my instructions and encouragement. And as
the week progressed, I asked him to read this message to the
entire team: "Thanks all for the love and support. Could not
do this alone."

Our quarterback, Andrew Luck, had told me how much he benefited from the Friday morning quarterback meetings he and I had prior to my illness. So I saw no reason to stop now. Andrew later told me, "When you walked us through ten or fifteen plays of the opposing defense, I learned a lot. But then with the leukemia, I figured we wouldn't be doing those meetings anymore, at least for a while. But on that first Friday before the Packers game, I received eight text messages from you — looks, indicators, and things to watch for."

I wanted the team and every person in the organization to know just how grateful I was to be a part of our big Colts family. When adversity strikes, families pull together, and I was experiencing the loving benefit of that support first-hand. I desperately wanted to be there in the locker room and on the sideline, but because that was impossible, I asked Bruce to read this letter to the team before the game against the Packers:

Dear Colts family,

On behalf of the Pagano family, we want to say thank you for all the love and support you have shown. We can never repay you, but just know that we love you all and we will always have your backs. We could not get through this without all of you!

All the cards, notes, texts, and emails have been read and digested. It's overwhelming. But right on time.

We will all be better in the long run. Thanks to all the survivors and your personal stories. They are truly inspiring. I know I will beat this, and hearing all the special success stories make the days much better!

You know I am going crazy in here, but nobody understands process better than all of us Colts.

My condition will not determine my position. I understand the condition, but choose to focus on my position. That is to stay positive and SERVE.

WE WILL! WE CAN! WE MUST! WE HAVE NO CHOICE. BY ANY MEANS NECESSARY. WE WILL OVERCOME.

IT'S ALL IN THE PROPER STATE OF MIND.

Know there is no better owner in the NFL, period! He has built an organization based on Faith, Family, and Football. Don't ever mistake the ORDER.

We all have a job to do. We know and understand that. That's why we signed up for it. We knew there were going to be tough times. This is not for everybody, but I know deep in my heart we are all here because we're supposed to be.

Focus on being .500 by 4:30 p.m. on Sunday. Nothing else. LASER-SHARP FOCUS. That has to be our mind-set.

Sixty minutes, all you got, one play at a time. Don't judge! WIN!

Respectfully,

Coach P

U

By the end of the week I was as sick as a dog, and I was upset that for the first time in practically my entire life I would not be on a football field, coaching. Football was as much a part of every fall as hayrides, bonfires, Halloween, and Thanksgiving. It's what I had done every fall since I played Pop Warner football, junior and high school football, and college football and then began coaching football. Now for the first time, I was sidelined, and it was beyond depressing!

One bright spot occurred when Mr. Irsay discovered that I had limited viewing options in my hospital room, and so he had NFL Network installed. Throughout my battle with cancer, I was consistently reminded how fortunate I am to have Jim Irsay as my friend, as the owner of the franchise, and as our leader.

In an interview that week, Mr. Irsay commented to the media, "Chuck is very dear to this organization. The special thing about Chuck is he's a salt-of-the-earth man. He's going to be greatly missed in terms of his intensity, his energy, his leadership — the things that made him the guy Ryan and I selected as our head coach. Chuck has had the chance three or four weeks into the season to set the tone for the coaches and the players. And meeting with the team, meeting with the coaches, there's nothing more we want than to have a victory ball from our Green Bay game, to walk into the hospital and put it in his hands."

His words not only lifted my spirits, but that of the entire organization as well. I truly cannot say enough good things about Mr. Irsay. There isn't a better person in the NFL.

A lot has been said about the strong loyalty that makes today's Colts a great team, and I'm the first to tell you it starts at the top of the organization with our owner. From the minute I met him and shook his hand, I knew he was a man of character. In getting to know him, I saw that the most important things to him are his faith, his family, and football. I can't begin to tell you how supportive he's been to my family and me. His loyalty and support permeate throughout the organization, and this is what makes our team so special. As we approached time for kickoff that Sunday afternoon, I was reminded yet again of his kindness and generosity.

∪

Bruce and I were concerned about how the players would react during the game. Would they play like a team with a higher purpose and overachieve to beat the favored Packers? Or would their concern with my health issues become a distraction and a drain on them emotionally? With this in mind, Bruce told them, "Don't play with too much emotion. Don't try to do more than you're capable. Don't try to do two jobs — doing your own job will suffice."

"One thing we have to do is be very aware of not getting overly excited or overly hyped about trying to do something extra," he said. "We can't get caught up in the snot bubbles and tears. They don't beat anybody. We're going to man up. Chuck would want it that way. We're going out there to win. We're going to make sure we continue to win so Chuck can be on the sideline with us in our first playoff game." That was the team's goal from day one.

Professional athletes are very good at compartmentalizing. They're able to put personal issues to the side when it's time to perform. When personal tragedy happens, a football player must be focused on his job — tackling, blocking, running, passing. When he's thinking about his assignments, he isn't thinking about anything else that could distract him.

"You try to put it aside a bit, as cold as that sounds," Andrew Luck, our rookie quarterback, said before the Green Bay game. "Our thoughts are with him in terms of everything we do. We break it down after practice on 'Chuck.' A lot of guys will be playing for him for a lot of games to come. But Coach will be disappointed if we're not putting full effort into practice or if we're getting too emotional about this situation."

U

With the hospital bed tilted up, I was in a semi-sitting position while Tina sat on the edge of the bed next to me. We were watching the pregame show, anxiously waiting for the kick-off. The cameraman scanned the stadium and zoomed in on a huge banner that read, "CHUCKSTRONG." Then another one appeared behind the opposite goalpost. Each banner was wrapped in a large orange ribbon. I don't know how the Colts' marketing department did it, but we saw thousands of fans wearing CHUCKSTRONG T-shirts. We were amazed to see the fans' support, and even more, we were happy to see how they were supporting the fight against leukemia. It brought us to tears.

We were also touched to see our guys wearing CHUCK-STRONG T-shirts during the warm-ups before the game. Even the Packers' players were wearing CHUCKSTRONG T-shirts when they warmed up. Evidently a lot of people bought T-shirts that Sunday, because the Colts donated $90,000 from sales to leukemia research.

Once the game started, Tina started screaming, hollering, and moving all over the place. During a commercial I looked at her and said, "Really? Is this how it's going to be for the next three hours and five minutes? Is this how you act when I'm on the field and you're up in the stands?" We laughed, but it was definitely a new experience for both of us.

Tina grew up as a football fan. Her three brothers played football, and her father coached their Little League teams. And in high school, Tina was a cheerleader. But I can't remember the last time we watched a game together. Any game I was involved in since we met, I was always coaching on the sideline and never with her. She'd either be in the stands or watching the game on television.

The sports commentator talked about the support the community and the team were giving us. He mentioned that the Colts' players were wearing CHUCKSTRONG T-shirts, and again our tears flowed. When Reggie Wayne entered the game, the camera zoomed in on Reggie and his bright orange gloves. When he lifted his arms and waved, the crowd roared its support and approval. Tina and I were overwhelmed once again.

U

The Packers were favored to roll over us. They had gone 15 – 1 during the regular season in 2011, and were one of only three teams in NFL history to score more than 35 points in nine games in a single season. Their quarterback, Aaron Rodgers, was considered among the best in the game. By the half, we were down 21 – 3, and it looked like the Packers were on their way to another 35-point game.

Still, our guys refused to allow the score to get them down. Later I discovered that during the halftime break, they recalled how we had bounced back from our previous losses. They began getting fired up to change the dynamic on the field. Cory Redding told his teammates, "We've *got* to win this thing. We can do it. Think about what Coach is going through. We gotta do this, guys!" With the same brand of fierce determination, Bruce reminded the team to stick to the process. "One play at a time," he emphasized. "Football games are won one play at a time. Don't get stuck in the last play. Don't jump ahead. One play at a time." Reggie Wayne added, "C'mon guys, we don't want to disappoint Chuck!"

Whatever the message was, it worked. After halftime, our guys took the field determined to play better and stick to the process. We kicked off to Green Bay, got them in a third-down situation, and intercepted the ball in Packers territory. Our offense scored a couple plays later, and the comeback was on. Then, midway through the third quarter, Adam Vinatieri booted a 50-yard field goal to make it 21 – 13. We were back within striking distance.

With 18 seconds left in the third quarter, Andrew Luck darted in from 3 yards out to bring us within two points, 21 – 19. We went for two points but didn't get it. However, early in the fourth quarter, Vinatieri kicked a 28-yard field goal, giving us our first lead of the game, 22 – 21. But after the kickoff, the Packers' Alex Green broke a 41-yard run on the first play, and with 4:30 minutes left in the game, Aaron Rodgers tossed an 8-yard TD pass that gave the Packers a 27 – 22 lead. They went for the two-point conversion, but we stopped them cold. Rodgers was clearly having a great game, completing 21 of 33 passes for 243 yards, with three touchdowns and one interception.

But our rookie quarterback wasn't doing so bad himself. After the kickoff, he led a fantastic drive down the field, completing third-down passes to Reggie Wayne, and on another third-down play, he scrambled for the first down to keep the drive going. Then, with 39 seconds left in the game, it was first and goal from the 4-yard line. Andrew dropped back to pass, stepped up, hit Reggie with a strike, just short of the end zone, and watched him stretch out to break the plane of the goal line. We went for two points and made it — we were up 30 – 27! The Packers took the kickoff and marched up the field, giving their kicker, Mason Crosby, a 52-yard shot at a field goal with 3 seconds to go. He missed the kick, and the game was over. Colts 30, Packers 27. We won! Our team turned the game around and refused to accept defeat.

They played like a great team and won like a great team. Now this was Colts football! Everyone played like a champion, and I was so proud of them. Andrew passed for 362 yards and broke the rookie quarterback single-game franchise record for the most passing yards. After the game he told a reporter, "We all went out there wanting to do it for Chuck more than anything else. To see all the emotions on Mr. Irsay's face, Bruce's, everyone there, I think it's one of the greatest athletic accomplishments I've ever been part of."

Reggie caught 13 passes for a career-high 212 yards and scored the game-winning TD. It was the second-highest receiving total in Colts history, behind Hall of Famer Raymond Berry's performance in 1957. It was also Reggie's 100th consecutive game with a catch. After the game, Reggie said, "Chuck instilled a lot in us. His whole motto since day one, the first meeting, has been team, team, team. Nothing else. So we've wanted to do it every week as a team. That's all we practice; that's all we preach."

A couple of hours after the game, I called Reggie. "My man, way to go," I said. "That's why I called you this summer. That's why I wanted you to take the leap of faith!"

"Man, how are you doing?" Reggie asked.

"I'm good," I answered.

I'm told that Mr. Irsay choked up when he addressed the team inside the locker room after the game. After his speech, Mr. Irsay rushed out of the room so he could personally deliver the game ball to me. I can't express in words how much his thoughtfulness meant to me. While many game balls have significance over the years, that one will always be extra special to me.

U

A few days after the Packers game, I received a call from my good friend Kevin Elko. Elks and I go way back to my six years with the Miami Hurricanes starting in 1995. Coach Butch Davis had frequently brought in Kevin to give inspirational talks to the team.

When Elks heard about my leukemia diagnosis, he called to ask, "What can I do for you?"

"You can pray for me," I said.

"Chuck, you know that's a given," he answered.

The next morning, I received the first of many "pep talks" Elks sent me:

> Hey, Chuck. You know how much I'm hurting with you over this. But you also know we're going to beat this. In John 15:1, Christ said to his disciples, "I am the true vine, and my Father is the vinegrower. He removes every branch in me that bears no fruit. Every branch that bears fruit he prunes to make it bear more fruit."
>
> Christ's half brother James tells us to be glad for our adversity, to be glad for our suffering. It will teach us patience, endurance, and how to do long-suffering.
>
> To get close to God, you must get into the things that he's into. And God is into the poor, the suffering, the lonely, and the sick. You will understand these things better now. Chuck, you were always kind. I remember back in '99 when Miami's standout safety Al Blades was killed in a car crash. It was two years after he left the Hurricanes to play for the 49ers. You were

the one who picked up the phone and called his teammates. You told them you loved them, and told them to be careful.

Yes, you were always kind, but now you will be kind in a different way than before. You will be more drawn to the sick. I remember when you once asked me, "Hey, Elks, I'm going to talk to somebody who's dying. What do I say?" Chuck, you will have a lot more of those calls now, and you will know what to say. You will have words to say now. Why? Because you have been pruned. Because you have gone through long-suffering, and God will be there with you. That's how you do it.

I had a friend who was my teammate when we were defensive backs in high school. Charlie was a wild kid. He got a virus that attacked the outer sheath of his spinal cord. He was in rehab in Morgantown, West Virginia. I walked into this room, and there was nothing to him. They had to pick him up and move him, and he was screaming. They put Charlie in a wheelchair, and he ordered me, "Wheel me down to the cafeteria." On the way, he spotted a woman in her nineties, and he said, "Stop." Charlie looked at her and said, "Who da man?" She said, "You da man." I could tell they'd gone through this routine before. He motioned to me to continue wheeling him down the hall. Charlie was having his own health problems, and yet he took time to be kind to this elderly woman. Through his pruning, he was closer to God.

Chuck, you are going to come out of this battle—and you will come out of it victorious—and when you do, you will be closer to God. You will be drawn to helping people more than you have ever been. I know you've always been a kind person, maybe even the kindest person I know. But you will be still kinder. The tree will be pruned, and when it is pruned, it will bear fruit. You were selected to be pruned. And you are going to be different than you ever were.

Love you,

Elks

Elks's pep talk really touched me. I knew what he said came straight from the heart. It made me start to think about how I could use my cancer to serve others. It helped me begin imagining what my life would be like — not *if* but *when* I beat cancer. I felt something growing inside me, the first stirrings of the greatest weapon we have against cancer: *hope.*

CHAPTER 6

STICK TO IT

Why We Lost to the Jets

How long should you try? Until.

—Jim Rohn

The Monday morning edition of the *Indianapolis Star* reported that our nail-biting upset over the Packers was the most emotional game ever played in the history of Lucas Oil Stadium. Whether or not that's true, I doubt anyone became more emotional than Tina and I did as we watched the game in my hospital room. It seemed like everyone in Indianapolis — no, in the country — watched the game.

Many former players, assistant coaches, and other football colleagues reached out to me after we beat the Packers. They wanted to contribute to the CHUCKSTRONG campaign, to let me know they were thinking of me and praying for me and my family, and to see if there was anything we needed. You never really realize how much others care until you're flat on your back and feeling lonely and discouraged. There's no time for self-pity, however, when so many people gather around to fight with you.

I had little energy and was weak. I felt tired from not being able to sleep at night. Plus, I was feeling the miserable side effects caused by my chemotherapy. Still I was alert and excited about our comeback win over the Packers, and we now had a 2 – 2 record.

Although I know there are no easy games in the NFL, we were feeling good about our upcoming game against the New York Jets in East Rutherford, New Jersey, on the next Sunday. The Jets were struggling offensively and had gotten beat the previous Sunday. They were 2 – 3 for the season. The Colts enjoyed a 40 – 29 lead in the overall series between the two teams and had won seven out of the last ten games. We were a three-point favorite; this was a game we felt we could win. However, as my cancer experience testified, events don't always go as planned.

U

Because you can't always count on life — or football games — to go as you expect, you have to focus on the process, do the work, take it one day at a time or one play at a time, and stick to it. For seven months before the season began, we talked to the team about how there are approximately 160 total plays in every game. We continually emphasized the process and the importance of playing hard on every play: "There are probably five or six out of those total plays that determine the outcome of a game. Most of the time, you are sparring with your opponent. You don't know which of those plays will determine if we win. So you keep playing and giving every play everything you got. Then when *that* play shows up, you're there to make it."

To get this point across, we showed a video of legendary Pittsburgh Steelers' running back Franco Harris's reception in the 1972 AFC divisional playoff game against the Oakland Raiders. The Raiders had scored a touchdown on a 30-yard run by quarterback Ken Stabler with 1:17 to go in the game and were up 7 – 6. With no time-outs remaining, the Steelers were facing a fourth and 10 on their own 40-yard line with only 22 seconds left on the clock. Under enormous pressure from Oakland's pursuing defensive linemen, Steelers quarterback Terry Bradshaw heaved the ball to the Raiders' 35-yard line toward his halfback, John Fuqua, who had it on his fingertips. The Raiders' hard-hitting safety Jack Tatum collided with Fuqua and knocked him to the ground, a sure incomplete pass as the ball went sailing backward, end over end, in the air.

Fullback Franco Harris's assignment was to block for his quarterback and then run downfield in the event Bradshaw needed another receiver. Just before the ball hit the ground, Harris managed to scoop it up while a Steelers tight end blocked a Raiders lineman. Harris used a stiff-arm to ward off a Raiders defensive back and barreled in for a touchdown with 5 seconds to go. The Steelers won the game 13 – 7. Myron Cope, a Pittsburgh sportscaster, dubbed it "the Immaculate Reception," and ever since, this incredible play has been known by this name. It's considered the greatest football play of all time. After the game, Franco Harris said, "I was just playing hard and giving it all I had."

I love his work ethic and how it paid off in such a dramatic way. Had Franco Harris been loafing, had he taken that play off, the ball would have fallen incomplete — and who knows where that franchise would be today. Just keep going hard at what you are doing. This has to be your mind-set for the entire game. There is going to be some sparring, and there will be some setbacks. Just make sure you are going hard, so you are there and ready.

I believe the Immaculate Reception was a critical turning point for the Steelers organization. For four previous decades the franchise had never won a playoff game. The Steelers went on to win four Super Bowls by the end of the 1970s. I remain convinced that with the same philosophy and commitment, we can do the same.

∪

Ever since my cancer diagnosis, Reggie Wayne and I had been constantly texting, emailing, and talking on the phone, and he kept asking when he could stop by to see me. That Tuesday after the Packers game, I asked him to visit me. Knowing that Reggie had lost some family members to leukemia, I suspected he was taking my cancer diagnosis very hard. So I wanted him to see for himself that I was alive and still kicking. Although he came to cheer me up, my plan was to make him feel better.

When Reggie walked into my room, he didn't know what to expect. He was wearing a mask because my doctors were worried that my immune system wouldn't be able to ward off germs and they wanted to keep me in a sterile environment. I was also wearing a mask. Even with a mask on, I could tell from Reggie's eyes that he didn't like what he saw. I had lost a lot of weight. I was weak. My hair was beginning to fall out. It was evident that cancer had taken a toll on me.

"Hey, Reggie," I greeted him as he entered my room. "Come in and grab a seat."

He was quiet and was at a loss for words, which is unusual for Reggie. The first thing I said to him was, "We're going to win this one."

"I believe you, Chuck."

Later Reggie described his first hospital visit and said, "When I heard Chuck tell me we were going to win, I knew he was going to be okay. I didn't need to cry anymore."

Reggie noticed I was working on my iPad on the table beside my bed. I had been looking at films of practices that Ryan routinely sent to me, and I began asking Reggie a lot of questions. I wanted details about how everyone was doing, how practice was going, who was banged up — all the little details that often told me so much. Reggie didn't like it at first, saying, "Chuck, what are you doing? You're supposed to be in here resting."

"This *is* my rest," I told him. "This is my healing."

"I didn't come here to talk about football," he said. "I came to see how you were doing."

"I can't wait to get out of here," I said. "I can't wait."

Tina walked in as Reggie and I were finishing our conversation, and he got up to give her a hug. "You should see how the two of you look," she said with a smile, "sitting there, talking to each other with those masks on! How can you even understand each other?"

When Reggie got up to say good-bye, he said to me, "Chuck, I'm feeling a thousand times better than I did before I walked into this room." He gave me a hug and walked out with a smile on his face. It had been great to see Reggie.

That week Reggie told a reporter, "I sat with him for a little while, and he's doing good, man. I was kind of surprised to see how good he was. He's the same. He was joking. He's looking at it straight now. He understands what's going on. He understands the tough task ahead of him. If there's anybody who can go in and hit this out of the ballpark, it's him."

Like I said, Reggie and I are close, and the other players knew we were tight, so they kept asking him, "How's Coach doing?" When I texted him, he'd sometimes read my texts at team meetings, and when we talked, Reggie would relay our conversations to the other players. "They keep asking me about your progress," Reggie told me. "These guys really worry about you, Coach."

I was touched by their concern. I am sure everyone's sentiments would have been the same for any member of our team. This is the family spirit we instilled in the team before the season began. I was happy to see everyone pulling together and heading in the same direction. This is what families do when they face adversity. When bad things happen, instead of folding, strong teams, like strong families, are galvanized and go on to do great things, such as winning championships. In the case of the Colts, we were determined to keep moving on to do the things nobody thought we could do.

U

Cory Redding was another one of the first players to visit me at the hospital. Like Reggie and me, Cory and I had been texting back and forth practically every day. When he walked into my room, he noticed I had a dry erase board on the wall with a depth chart on it. I was walking around in my room and started talking football with him. I asked him a lot of questions about the guys, and I gave him some instructions to pass along to other players. This was my way of letting Cory know he shouldn't be worrying about me.

Cory is a very spiritual man, and while he was visiting me, we prayed together, which was good for both of us. I love what Cory said to the media: "The Super Bowl is what we always talk about. That's on his list. And I want to scratch it off with him. As a friend first and as a player second, I'm going to do everything in my power to help make that happen."

During Cory's visit he reminded me of what we had been repeating to the team since the day we came to Indianapolis: "From the time you arrived here, Chuck," he said, "you embodied that we are here to serve one another. That was one of the main things you said on the first day we all came together as a team in training camp. You told us, 'We are here to serve, and that means on the field and off the field. Sacrifice. Give everything you've got for the man next to you, your brother, because he will do the same for you.' I took those words very seriously, Coach, and I try to live by them every day."

When Cory said this to me, I knew if he and Reggie were understanding and demonstrating what it meant to love their teammates like brothers, this mind-set of sacrificial servant-hood would be picked up by other players and permeate throughout the organization. It was great to see Cory.

∪

Many people have asked how I could've bonded with the Colts' organization and my players in such a short amount of time. I don't have an answer, other than to say that we believed in each other. We tried to demonstrate trust, loyalty, and respect in how we conducted ourselves with every single person in our organization. We needed to see these three intangibles in action if we were going to believe in them and practice them.

One of the first guys I met when I started working at the Colts' facility was a custodian named Angel. Every day he worked hard and demonstrated enthusiasm, commitment, and excellence. He loved to serve, and it showed. One day I invited Angel to join us for a player meeting. I introduced him to the guys and then asked if anyone knew his role in our organization. The veteran players knew Angel, and the newcomers quickly learned. They could tell I was not patronizing Angel, but that I genuinely appreciated and cared about him in the same way I cared and appreciated them. We were all in this together, and that was the only way we would ever win and sustain a great team.

With this conviction in mind, I like to think our players' support for me while battling leukemia was the same support we would show for any member of our Colts family facing something of this magnitude. They knew I'd do the same for them. They knew I needed them in order to win my fight and get back on the field with them. We all need each other. No man is better than any other. We each have our roles and must give all we've got to lift our team.

That's how I see coaching. When you're dealing with these men, if they believe all you want to do is use them as tools to win games and that's all that matters to you, they're not going to give you much loyalty. But if you really care about them as human beings, that's much different. Of course, I do want my players to succeed on the field, but maybe even more important, I want them to be good people and succeed off the field too. Character always matters, no matter whether you're in a boardroom or on a football field, in a cubicle or on a construction site. When people know you genuinely care about them, they will reward you with their confidence, trust, and belief. I never forgot what veteran NFL coach Dick Vermeil told me a long time ago: "People don't care how much you know until they know how much you care." I think that's a great statement — one I totally adhere to.

We all know what the expectations are in this league, and everybody knows we are judged on one thing — wins and losses. I want to win as much as anybody, but we can't place all of our emphasis on that and drop the ball on everything else. Our approach at the Colts is to accentuate the human side of the equation. I believe my role as the head coach is to assemble a group of men who trust each other and who understand the value of building strong relationships. Taking care of each other and having each other's backs are top priorities around here.

It's true we share a common goal with the other thirty-one NFL teams, and we, too, chase it every day. We are here to win games and claim championships. However, we're going to do it by building on a foundation of trust, loyalty, and respect. If your locker room is not united, you have no chance in this league. I don't care how good your players are. If there is a dysfunction in your team relationships, you'll have distractions, and your team is in trouble. The team dynamics on the field begin long before kickoff.

When we enter this building, players and coaches alike understand our priorities. Then when we're away from here, we pick up our lives again. There, too, we're together. We help each other. The human element is stressed in this organization. We understand everyone has issues off the field. We all have families, kids, relationships — and this is all part of it. We are all here together, helping each other navigate through the time we have together on this planet.

My relationships with players, coaches, franchise executives, and other staff members are extremely important. To me, going after our ultimate goal without building that bond would be meaningless. Naturally, you need great players. Every franchise needs exceptional athletes on the playing field. And keep in mind that in this game, whether it's in high school, college, or the NFL, it's hard to win at any level without a strong quarterback. You've got to have talented players to win consistently, and you've got to have them working together as a team. Having said this, to win championship after championship, you must have guys who care for one another and who are willing to sacrifice for each other. This is key.

U

Throughout my stay in the hospital, team owner Jim Irsay regularly stopped by to say hello and see how I was doing. His genuine concern went beyond my simply being his head coach. He cared for me as though I were a member of his family. I later found out he made many calls to Larry Cripe, my oncologist, checking on my status, wanting to know firsthand how I was doing. With my full consent, Dr. Cripe kept Mr. Irsay informed on a regular basis. In turn, Mr. Irsay gave updates on my health status to the team. Before our game with the Packers, he stated unequivocally to the team, "We are going to beat the Packers, and afterward I will take the game ball to Chuck in the hospital. Then we are going to extend the season, so Chuck can coach the team at the time when he'll be cleared by his doctors."

During my stay in the hospital, I also was in constant contact with our general manager, Ryan Grigson. Having an iPad during my stay in the hospital was a godsend. It kept me in touch with what was going on every day with the team. Ryan made sure films of the practices were delivered daily to me, and in this modern age of technology I was able to observe what was happening on the practice field while confined to my hospital room. I could regularly communicate with the players and coaches by means of text messages, emails, and telephone calls. Although I wasn't there in the flesh, technology kept me connected with everyone.

Ryan and I had become friends before I became sick, and interestingly, our bond grew even stronger during my illness. Ryan attributes it to the fact that we share the same core values and speak a similar language. "It's not just our beliefs regarding football," he points out, "but it also has to do with life in general." Ryan says my illness put things in perspective for him. "The personal relationships are what really matter in life," he says. "It's not money or wins."

Like me, Ryan raves about Mr. Irsay's support when I became sick. "Jim was like a rock," he said. "He was so positive about Chuck beating cancer and getting well that he energized me to pick myself up by the bootstraps and help lead the organization at a critical time. Right from the start, Jim put everything in a strong perspective, and from that point on, I just followed his lead. It was my first year as a general manager, and he made it clear to me that I had to be the backbone of this organization during this unbelievably difficult time for all."

Then it was Bruce Arians — or B.A., as we call him — who stepped in for me, and like Mr. Irsay, he constantly emphasized to the team, "We are going to win and extend the season, so Chuck can be on the sideline as our coach in the playoffs." Bruce made it crystal clear to the team that he was not replacing me — he was an interim coach who was sitting in for me until my health was restored.

No matter how absorbed B.A. was in his daily duties as head coach during my absence, first and foremost on his mind was the reality that his friend was fighting a battle in the hospital. He was always saying to the players, "Hey, man, don't feel sorry for yourselves. I don't care if you are hurting right now. Somebody out there is in worse condition than you are. Remember why we're doing this. Don't forget about Chuck."

I'm told that B.A. never addressed the team without mentioning my name and reminding them what they were playing for. "I am looking forward to the day," he always emphasized, "when Chuck is back, and he can take back the torch he passed to me." I can't think of a better example of true friendship and selflessness than what B.A. displayed. He exemplified our philosophy of caring for each other and covering each other's back. Bruce truly walked the talk, and by doing so, he distinguished himself as an outstanding leader. There is no doubt the players picked up on the loyalty and dedication he showed to me. By his actions, he was demonstrating to them what they should do for each other.

U

Our game against the Jets approached. Even though we were playing on the road, they had lost their last two home games, so it looked like momentum was on our side. Our outside linebackers, Robert Mathis and Dwight Freeney, were injured, but the Jets would be playing without All-Pro cornerback Darrelle Revis, and their wide receiver Santonio Holmes was out for the season. Their quarterback, Mark Sanchez, was struggling with a 48.4 percent pass completion rate in their first four games, and rumors continued to swirl that head coach Rex Ryan might replace him with Tim Tebow.

The Jets had acquired Tebow from Denver in a highly publicized off-season trade, and he had been used sparingly, mainly as a running quarterback to throw opponents off guard. Prior to our game, he had 57 yards on 14 runs and 7 yards in the air on two attempts. The Jets' offense was struggling, ranking near the bottom of the league in yards per game. Again, this was a game where it appeared we should win. But one thing you learn pretty quickly in football — just as we experienced with the Jaguars, anything can happen.

U

And it did. The game started off slowly, with both teams moving the ball back and forth without scoring. With 6 minutes to go in the first quarter, we scored on a 20-yard field goal by Adam Vinatieri. The quarter ended 3 – 0.

Then less than a minute into the second quarter, Mark Sanchez completed a 5-yard TD pass to Stephen Hill, and the Jets went ahead 7 – 3. Their Shonn Greene scored on a 10-yard run in the middle of the quarter, and with 6 minutes left in the half, Adam Vinatieri added three points to our score with a 50-yard field goal. Then on a fourth and 11 from the Colts' 40, Tebow, aligned in his normal position as the personal protector, took a direct snap, threw a jump pass to a linebacker, which resulted in a 23-yard gain. The play brought the home crowd to its feet with a loud cheer for the newly acquired backup quarterback. With 27 seconds to go in the half, Sanchez fired another 5-yard touchdown pass, giving the Jets a 21 – 6 lead going into the locker room.

It got worse in the second half. Simply put, it wasn't our best half of football. We weren't playing Colts football, and the Jets dominated the game. Sanchez completed 11 of 18 passes for only 82 yards, but two of those passes went for touchdowns. We were unable to stop their ground game. Their running back Shonn Greene had a career-high 161 yards on 32 carries and three touchdowns, and the Jets amassed 252 yards on the ground. They averaged 5.7 yards per rushing attempt, compared to our 2.4 yards per carry. Sadly, even though we knew the Jets' game plan was to run the ball, we still couldn't stop them.

The Jets were 5 for 5 in the red zone, the area from the defense's 20-yard line to the end zone where scoring most frequently happens, compared to our 0 for 2. Offensively, we completed 22 of 44 passes for 280 yards, but we threw two interceptions and fumbled away the ball on one play. The Jets sacked Andrew Luck four times, bringing his total to 17 sacks in five games.

B.A. summed up our performance against the Jets this way: "If you can't block and you can't tackle, you can't win. It's the fundamentals, the things we identified going into the game — fake punts, stopping the run, protecting the quarterback. Red zone offense and defense were keys to the game. We didn't win in any of those areas."

∪

The following Monday morning, I woke up discouraged and already exhausted before the day began. But then I received a friendly reminder about the power of faith in this voice mail message left by Kevin Elko:

Chuck, now that we know what's going on with your diagnosis, the first quarter is over. We are going into the second quarter, and now is a good time to talk about having faith.

Faith is believing in things you have not seen. Your reward is that by having faith, you get to see it. There was a time when I didn't realize that faith is an intentional thing. I thought that the separation of the Red Sea was a miracle, but I had never experienced a miracle. I later came to realize that miracles constantly come my way. Most people don't have faith and are unable to understand that faith is intentional. Each of us has to make a decision that he wants to be a person of faith. It's just that easy. You just make that decision.

Again, you have to believe in things you have not seen. For example, in our economy, we trade in paper, and we spend money to acquire possessions. But this is not how God's economy works. In his economy, we trade in faith. Every single time Christ healed somebody, he had one phrase — "Go and sin no more" — but people misinterpret this quote. When Christ healed the sick and they'd say, "Thank you; you healed me," he said, "No, your faith healed you." Chuck, I have talked to people who are healed from cancer, and I discovered they are never shocked by it. I repeat, being cured from cancer didn't shock them.

Lee Ford, my neighbor, was crossing the street and got hit by a car going forty miles an hour. They gave him an hour to live. They then said Lee would live for twenty-four hours. Then they said he'd be dead in a week. After that they said he would live, but he'd be a quadriplegic and blind. Then that prognosis was changed. He would just be blind. Lee is now fully recovered. It just took a while. I talked to him about it, and he said, "My wife left me, and I married Meredith, a wonderful woman. We had a child with Down syndrome. My wife and child needed me. Kevin, I believed in spite of the evidence, and then I watched the evidence change. God doesn't want you to say you have faith; he wants you to show it. You know God parted the sea twice for the Israelites. The first time he did it for Moses. Then it happened to Joshua. The rabbis with him were carrying the ark of the covenant, and they had to have the sea separate. God made them get down in it. They were walking, and the water was up to their knees. This wasn't like before. They started looking at God. "What's going on?" they asked. They were told, "Keep walking." They had to show God they had faith. God wants to see if you have faith, Chuck. He wants to see if you believe in your tools.

When David was getting ready to fight Goliath, King Saul tried to give him some armor. David said, "I don't need your armor. I don't need your spears. I have faith in my tools. I have faith in this small rock. I don't need what you offer me."

God wants to see if you have faith in your treatment. He said, "My son didn't just believe in it; he did it." Faith is believing in things you have not seen, and it's about the reward you get. God wants to see if you have faith in him and in the plan he has for your life.

In Jeremiah 29:11, it is written, " 'I know the plans I have for you,' declares the Lord." Chuck, God has a plan for you. I have complete faith at my end. I have faith in you and in our Maker. I have faith in everything that surrounds you.

I hope you feel better today. Talk to you later.

CHAPTER 7

THREE STRAIGHT WINS

The Best Homecoming Present

Adversity causes some men to break,
others to break records.

—William Arthur Ward

By the second week of chemo, my hair started falling out. One day when I got up to go to the bathroom, Tina and I noticed my hairs on the pillow. It wasn't like it all came out in big chunks — just lots of loose hairs everywhere. I told her I felt like I was shedding more than our dog. Some of my friends might have said I didn't have any hair to spare in the first place. But it was just one more sign that this was my reality.

So one day, I decided just to embrace this new reality. Tina and I had fallen into a routine by then. After our devotional and prayer time, she'd get my breakfast and help me get settled. Then she would run home for a couple of hours to take a shower, do the laundry, walk the dog — all the things that needed to be done to keep us going. One morning while she was gone, one of the nurses came in to check my vitals and noticed all the hairs on my pillow. She said, "Looks like it's starting to go. What do you think — want me to get my clippers?"

The thought of being totally bald when Tina returned made me smile, so I nodded, and sure enough, the nurse came back in with an electric barber clipper. It probably only took about thirty seconds to get rid of the little hair I had left.

"There, that's better," she said as she began cleaning up the loose hairs with a towel. "It looks good on you. Bald men are sexy, right?"

I was too tired to argue or even make any kind of joke in response. When Tina walked in my room a little later, she didn't say anything right away, but I could tell she noticed.

"When did you find time to go to the barbershop?" she asked, half teasing.

I told her about the nurse.

My wife ran her hand across my bare scalp and said, "She did a good job. You look great bald. Not every guy does, but it looks good on you. What do you think?"

"I'm going to shave it next year for training camp," I said. "Maybe I'll get the guys to do it with me."

"No, you're not," Tina replied, laughing. "You'll scare the crap out of every player on your team!"

U

I was officially allowed to have visitors, but usually only one or two at a time, and just for a few minutes. I loved seeing anyone from the Colts, but eventually the fatigue would catch up with me, and I'd barely be able to keep my eyes open. Since Dr. Cripe came in every day, he often got to meet my visitors. I remember one time several of the assistant coaches were visiting, and it was great. We sat around talking about the previous week's game, dissecting every play as they filled me in on all the sideline details. Dr. Cripe came in and met everyone, and the coaches immediately started asking him questions.

He's a patient man, and I could also tell he was amused by how persistent their questions were.

"So, Doc," Charlie Williams said, "how long before Coach can be back doing his job? You think he'll be ready by Thanksgiving?"

"As I've told Chuck, it's hard to say," answered Dr. Cripe.

"Well, can you give us a rough estimate — maybe a range of dates, you know, best case and worst case?" Charlie continued. "Maybe before the end of the season? Christmas?"

Laughing, Dr. Cripe said, "You guys — I wish I knew."

"Sorry," Charlie explained, "it's the way we operate. When

we have a goal, we have to set a date, break it down — you start wishing everything in life could be that way."

Later, Dr. Cripe told me that depending on whether my counts continued to climb, I might be able to go home soon and do the remaining two rounds as an outpatient. This gave me new incentive to stay positive, force myself to eat, and focus on being back in the game with my guys.

U

One of the hardest parts of being in the hospital was seeing other patients in far worse condition than me. Dr. Cripe and our nurses encouraged me to try to walk a little each day around the halls and get as much exercise as possible. They didn't want me going anywhere beyond my care center in the hospital since it was a sterile environment and my immune system remained weak.

Some days I didn't have the energy, and other days I just didn't want to be reminded of my confinement in a hospital. Strangely enough, it was easier to stay positive in my room because I could go over plays, text coaches and players, and talk on the phone. I could watch the games on my computer or iPad and think through plays for our remaining opponents. Even though it was still a hospital room, I could immerse myself in football and escape, at least for a while.

A few times, while on a walk in the hallway, Tina and I would stop to talk to another patient. One time a nurse told me about an older woman whose condition was terminal, and I made it a point to talk with her for a bit. I tried to encourage her, to ask about her family, to look for ways I could cheer her up. But it was hard. I didn't really know what to say. We stood there with our sterile breathing masks on, trying to be strong for each other.

As much as I wanted to help others beat cancer, I still had my own battle to fight. But I looked forward to the day when I would be strong enough to come back and encourage people. To let them know they've got to fight, to give them hope, to tell them they're not alone. This vision gave me one more reason to fight harder — I wanted to be able to help others beat cancer.

U

By the time we played the Cleveland Browns, I was able to watch it from my own home. Dr. Cripe held true to his promise, and because my counts continued to improve, he discharged me to go home. I still had two more rounds to complete before we would know if my cancer was in remission, but I would undergo those as an outpatient, visiting the hospital each day for a chemo treatment.

Being in my own home with Tina and watching my own TV screen made my life feel just a bit more like normal. I was still weak but excited to be back home. Now the best homecoming gift I could ask for would be a win over the Browns. Going into the game, our record stood at 2 – 3 on the season, so if we were to win this game, we'd already have won more games than the previous year.

When it was all said and done, Andrew Luck ran for two touchdowns, a testament to his mobility in the pocket and ability to scramble — he became the first Colts QB to score more than one running TD in a game in almost twenty-five years. It was a low-scoring game, but the guys played good football.

We were able to control the ball for over half the game, and we got our running game going for a season-high 148 yards. On the other hand, the Browns could not establish the run. This time our team didn't have to rally in the fourth quarter to come from behind. Later I found out Mr. Irsay had delivered a great postgame speech that really made the guys appreciate the win, knowing I was able to watch from home. I wasn't sure when it would be, but I just knew I would be back on the field before the season ended.

U

Our next game was on the road against the Tennessee Titans, and it didn't go quite as smoothly as our win over the Browns. We tied the Titans, each of us with a field goal, in the first quarter, but after that Tennessee led most of the game. Watching the game at home was frustrating. I kept yelling instructions, plays, and encouragement to our guys through the TV as if they could hear me.

Our defense kept us within striking distance, and our offense kept striking. The Titans sacked Andrew twice, grabbed an interception, batted down a couple passes, and blocked a 37-yard field goal attempt at the end of the first half. But they couldn't keep us from drilling the secondary and finding open receivers time and time again. Andrew led two 80-yard touchdown drives, including a 1-yard TD run by Delone Carter to tie the game at 13. We were still in this thing.

Our defense held them, and with the clock ticking down to zero, we were headed to overtime. Some coaches have special plays, formations, and systems just for overtime. While I understand their thinking, it's not my philosophy. I've always encouraged our players to stay focused on the next play, and then the next, whether it's the first quarter or the overtime period.

Football is all about the process. We had played for 60 minutes, and now we got a few more in overtime. But the basics stayed the same. You can only focus on the play you've got right now, so don't judge what's already happened. Don't look at the scoreboard and panic if you're trailing or coast if you're ahead. If you're up or down, just play your best one play at a time.

We stuck to this process every day of the week and didn't deviate because of a heartbreaking loss or an amazing win. When the players came in on Monday morning, I wanted them to know I would be the same guy with the same message, not Dr. Jekyll if we won and Mr. Hyde if we lost. It was going to be matter-of-fact — win or lose, we would take a look at the tape, point out the good things, identify the mistakes we made and the areas we need to correct, and focus on how we can move forward and get better as a team.

The message was simple: stick with the process. Ryan, Bruce, and our coaching staff had a few areas we wanted to pound home, week in and week out, and process was essential. Now against the Titans in overtime, that process was about to be tested.

Barely 5 minutes into overtime, Andrew connected with Vick Ballard on a little screen pass in the red zone. Ballard ran up the left alley toward the end zone when several Tennessee defenders converged to try to push him out of bounds. They knocked Vick's feet out from under him and sent him flying into the air like a pole vaulter trying to clear the bar. He crossed the goal line upside down, with his head hitting the pylon that marked the corner of the end zone.

Everyone held their breath as we awaited the official review … touchdown! With our 19 – 13 victory, the Indianapolis Colts now had a winning record of 4 – 3. Tina and I were ecstatic. I was hoping to be at the game the next week. I might not be ready to coach on the sideline yet, but I thought I was strong enough to attend the Dolphins game in person.

U

My counts were staying steady, so Dr. Cripe told me that if I didn't overdo it, I could attend the Miami game that week. After a week at home to rest, I would be starting the next round of chemo, which meant daily trips to the Simon Cancer Center. Although I wasn't sure how I'd feel by the end of the week, I was determined to be at the game that week, no matter what.

Mr. Irsay and Ryan were thrilled to hear I wanted to attend but wanted to be sure I was up for it. Tina let them know that, at this point, if I didn't get to go, my disappointment would be a bigger setback than my expending the energy to attend. They made sure Dr. Cripe was on board with the decision, knowing there would be extra media coverage at an already high-energy game. The last thing Mr. Irsay wanted was for my doctor to tune in to the game and be surprised to see me at a Colts game too soon.

The day of the game, I was like a little kid going to see his favorite team play for the first time. What a great feeling! It choked me up to be back at Lucas Oil Stadium. It felt like coming home.

Word spread quickly that I'd be attending and watching from up in the coaches' box with Ryan. I wanted to visit the locker room before the game. I wanted the team to see me and know I was beating this thing — that we would continue to beat it, together, as a family.

U

Games don't get any better than the one between the Colts and the Dolphins that Sunday afternoon. It had been so great to see the players, shake hands, say a few words, and let them know I was with them all the way. I reminded them about staying with the vision and not letting circumstances dictate their responses. It was such a moving time for all of us. I knew in my heart that we could win this game — that we *would* win this game — not because of me, but because we were a family. A family determined to win. A team united. A team that knew we would get the job done, by any means necessary.

The game couldn't have been more exciting. It was the kind of game where the teams appear to be evenly matched, and each one stays right with the other to keep up, like in a chess match. The game had been hyped all week because of the matchup between two outstanding rookie quarterbacks — our Andrew Luck and Miami's Ryan Tannehill.

Like gunslingers at a shooting range, these two young men showed just how good they are. In the first half, Andrew found Reggie Wayne in the south end zone from 9 yards out. Reminiscent of the Green Bay Packers' "Lambeau Leap," where a scoring player will leap up into the stands to receive pats, cheers, and high fives, Reggie jumped up above the CHUCK-STRONG banner to greet fans by slapping hands with his orange gloves, and they went wild. I was deeply moved to see so much support from the fans.

But the game was far from over. Tannehill and the Dolphins matched our score with an impressive 31-yard strike for a touchdown. But then Andrew came back on the field and completed a perfect pass down the middle for 48 yards! I was going nuts with the other coaches.

In the third quarter, we were trailing 17 – 13 when Andrew found T.Y. Hilton in the end zone with a laser-perfect pass thrown into double coverage. T.Y. made a spectacular leaping catch, and we now led the game by 3. It didn't take Miami long to tie it up, though, early in the fourth quarter. At that point, I wondered if this was going to be another overtime game, like the one we had with the Titans the week before. If it was going to have the same outcome, I wouldn't mind it.

But our team got it done without needing more than the 60 minutes of regulation playing time. With about 6 minutes left in the game, Andrew led our guys down the field, covering 69 yards in thirteen plays, to set up a 43-yard field goal by our veteran kicker, Adam Vinatieri. With plenty of time left on the clock, we knew Tannehill and the Dolphins could still score. It would be another test for our Colts defense.

Test passed. The defense held Miami in not one but two possessions. We got the ball back in the last couple minutes of the game, and Vick Ballard powered his way downfield for 19 yards, giving us a first down that would allow us to run out the clock and seal the victory. I had never been prouder of our team. Everyone fulfilled his role, did his job, and focused on the next play. We were playing like a team — not individuals — intent on winning.

U

With our record at 5 – 3, we now had won more than twice as many games as we had the prior season, in half the time. Andrew Luck had a monster game against Miami, throwing for 433 yards and two touchdowns, completing 30 of 48 passes, making good on 13 of 19 third-down conversions. He topped Cam Newton's NFL record of 422 yards, established in the previous season, for passing yards by a rookie quarterback.

And Andrew tied another record by becoming the NFL's second rookie QB to produce four 300+ yard games in a season. The other? His predecessor in Indianapolis — Peyton Manning. After the game, Andrew remained humble, praising his teammates and crediting my words before the game as the team's inspiration. He said, "Coach Pagano's presence is felt every day in the facility, but to see him in the flesh in the locker room, to hear him speak — it gave all the guys a boost."

Mr. Irsay asked me if I was up to going to the locker room to celebrate with the team, and I told him, "You couldn't keep me away!" When I entered, all the guys were simply going nuts, exchanging hugs and high fives. I can't tell you how good it felt to be back in that environment. With Bruce alongside me, I moved to the center of the locker room and knew what I wanted to say.

"I mentioned before the game that you guys were living in a vision and not living in circumstances," I said as players closed in around me to listen. "You know where they had us in the beginning, every last one of them. But you refused to live in circumstances, and you decided consciously, as a team and as a family, to live in a vision, and that's why you bring things home like what you brought home today. That's why you're already champions and well on your way."

I heard a few voices say "Amen!" and "Yessir!" as I continued.

"I've got circumstances. You guys understand it. I understand it. *It's already beat.* The vision that I'm living is to see two more daughters get married, dance at their weddings, and then hoist the Lombardi Trophy and watch that confetti fall on this group right here. Several times we're going to hoist that baby! I'm dancing at two more weddings, and we're hoisting that trophy together, men. Congratulations. I love all of you. Thank you — thank you all so much."

CHAPTER 8

BATTLE FATIGUE

Getting Sicker before Getting Better

Ability is what you're capable of doing.
Motivation determines what you do.
Attitude determines how well you do it.

—Lou Holtz

My talk with the team in the locker room after our win over Miami went viral and would later be nominated for the "Best Moment" Award at the 2013 ESPY Award ceremony. My words and the intensity of my emotion expressed the fighting spirit of so many men and women and boys and girls battling cancer. It made me incredibly happy to know that somehow the victory shared by me and the team could be extended to thousands of others in their own battles against cancer.

It also amazed me just how many people saw the video. My daughter Taylor called me later and told me a great story. She's attending medical school in Arizona, studying naturopathic medicine, which I know must have made it even harder for her to watch me as I went through chemotherapy. One day she walked into a class, and her professor began by telling the students, "I don't usually follow sports, but I have this story I want to tell you about." He then told the class about my speech.

Taylor sat there with a smile on her face, holding back a few tears. She didn't say anything then about being my daughter for the same reason she hadn't mentioned it to anyone before. She didn't want any kind of special treatment or, heaven forbid, for anyone to think she was remotely any kind of celebrity or related to one.

I've always told my kids that what I do is a job — a wonderful job that I love doing — but it's not who I am. I'm their dad. So I've always said not to make a big deal about being the daughter of a football coach. Just keep your head down and do the best you can at what you're supposed to be doing.

So Taylor just sat there in class without saying anything. She knew a couple of her friends knew — they had already figured it out because of her last name. But after class Taylor talked with her professor and told him that the paper she had turned in that week also recounted my speech in the locker room after the Dolphins game. He was simply stunned that Taylor was my daughter and was going through this journey with me and the rest of our family.

Sometimes it's a small world.

U

After the incredible win over Miami, we had a short week — only four days — until we played Jacksonville on the road in a Thursday night, prime-time matchup. It's always tough to play games back-to-back, with little time in between to rest and recover. Road games are tough as well, so when you put the two together, it adds an extra layer of difficulty.

Talking to Bruce, I know he shared my concern about whether the team would be ready to face the Jaguars again. We feared that after the incredible emotional high of the previous week's win, the team might feel spent, wiped out by the prospect of having to do the whole thing over again so quickly.

I toyed with the idea of going with the team but knew it was out of the question. As much as I had loved being at the Miami game, it took a lot out of me physically. I felt much weaker the next day, and I had to face resuming my own battle by returning to the chemo treatments. I didn't want to risk a setback by doing too much too soon. So I continued to review game tapes, text, call, and email Ryan, B.A., coaches, and players.

After the Jags pulled a last-minute win on us early in the

season, and considering how close some of our games had been — winning by three points or less, one game in over-time — I was more than a little worried. Coming into this game, Jacksonville had lost five in a row, so this was a big home game for them. They desperately needed a win, and having already beat us once, they would be gunning for us with a lot of confidence.

However, it was clear from the start that we were in command of the game. We scored on three consecutive possessions in the first half, jumping out to a 17 – 0 lead. Seeing the handwriting on the wall, many Jacksonville fans left at half-time, tired of losing so many games, with another loss almost in the books.

It was one of those games where nothing seemed to go the Jags' way. Their great running back Maurice Jones-Drew was out for a third straight game. Laurent Robinson fumbled at the end of a 9-yard gain, as our defender, Moise Fokou, stripped the ball from him. Officials first ruled Robinson was down, but the call was overturned on review, giving us possession.

This turnover led to our second touchdown, which clearly upset Jags' head coach Mike Mularkey. We drove down the field and ended up with a fourth and goal. Bruce decided to go for it, which is what I was shouting into my TV. Andrew kept the ball and ran it in. As our quarterback plunged over the cluster of linemen to cross the goal line, the ball appeared to be coming loose. Because all scoring plays are automatically reviewed, it took a couple minutes to get the ruling — touchdown!

A frustrated Coach Mularkey wanted officials to review it again because he was convinced Andrew had lost the ball. But because the play had already been reviewed, it wasn't open to further scrutiny, and so the officials ruled it couldn't be challenged. Coach Mularkey grabbed his headset and play sheet and threw them on the field, drawing a flag for unsportsmanlike conduct.

I've been there and know that feeling only too well. In his place, I might have done the same thing. When the game's not going your way, every single mistake or apparent injustice makes you crazy. One of the things that keeps me from losing it, though, is realizing the players are watching. Sure, the TV cameras are watching, as well as millions of fans. But I don't want the players to see me lose control and assume they can do the same thing. I really want to try to keep my composure, stay focused on the task at hand, make the necessary adjustments, and move on. In other words, I want to remind myself to *stick to the process.*

We went on to beat the Jags 27 – 10. Winning our fourth game in a row, we were now 6 – 3. Andrew Luck had a solid game, completing 18 of 26 passes, bouncing back after an interception and a fumble. But he couldn't be stopped in the red zone, using pump fakes and scrambling to keep defenders guessing. He ran 5 yards for a touchdown on one drive and then barreled across the goal line on a fourth-down play on the next possession.

The Colts had now won twice as many games as we'd lost on the season. Commentators and pundits were starting to include us on potential playoff lists. We were in the hunt.

U

In addition to our fourth straight win, I continued to be greatly encouraged by all the letters, emails, and gifts from so many fans, cancer survivors, and fellow fighters like myself still in the battle. I still remember how unbelievable the whole CHUCKSTRONG movement seemed to me. Once I overheard Tina talking on the phone with our youngest daughter, Tori, who was still in school back east. She's our little techie and always up on the latest technology and social media trends. Not long after I entered the hospital, she called Tina one day and said, "Did you know there's this whole CHUCKSTRONG campaign? There's even a Twitter account for it."

Tina asked, "What are you talking about?"

"There's even a website for it," Tori explained and gave her mom the address.

Tina and I were speechless. I really couldn't believe that so many people rallied around my battle with leukemia. But I remain thrilled to see the many positive outcomes emerging from the CHUCKSTRONG movement. I never wanted it to be about me, and honestly I felt a little uncomfortable about my name being front and center. In fact, I started adding the word *strong* to people's names whenever I thought they needed extra encouragement.

So I started calling my wife TINASTRONG, as well as using it with other friends and cancer patients I would talk to. It usually made them smile and reminded them that we're all in this battle together. No one person is more important than anyone else. I'm just a guy fighting cancer alongside the young kids, the soccer moms, the grandmothers — one of the more than fourteen million individuals diagnosed with this horrible disease each year.

When families are hit with adversity, everyone has to come together and share the load. They have to galvanize. I was experiencing it with my Colts family, but I was also experiencing it with my new, much larger extended family of people fighting cancer together.

As I became more and more worn-out from the fatigue brought on by my latest round of chemo, I remembered just how fortunate I was. The type of leukemia I had was a curable one. So many people on 3 East, my floor at the Simon Cancer Center, came in with diagnoses that meant they weren't leaving. As battle-fatigued as I was, I continued to be deeply grateful for all the love and support I had. And I continued to be so encouraged by the dramatic performance of our Colts team during the 2012 season.

No one thought we would even have a winning record this year, let alone be looking at making the playoffs. If a gambler had made a bet on the Colts with the oddsmakers before the season that we would be 6 – 3 going into week 10, they would have cashed in big. No one expected us to turn things around so quickly. No one knew for sure how good Andrew Luck would be as a rookie.

But I knew the season wasn't over yet. We still had seven games to play in the regular season. We had to keep our eyes on each game and not get carried away by assuming we'd get to where we wanted to be. Faith is crucial; action is essential. We had to stay humble, ignore the noise — good or bad — and keep working to get better every day.

U

After our Thursday night win over the Jags, we had ten days to prepare for one of the best teams in the league, the New England Patriots, who were led by future Hall of Fame quarterback Tom Brady, a gifted leader who had taken his team to the Super Bowl five times since being selected in the 2000 draft.

Under Brady's high-scoring offense, the Pats had won three of those five Super Bowl games, and he had been named the MVP for two of those victories. This season the Patriots once again seemed to be building momentum for the playoffs. They were the NFL's highest-scoring team and best offense. Their defense, however, was struggling, and this was where I hoped we'd have a chance of taking home the victory.

Another road game, this time in Foxborough, Massachusetts. It began with a back-and-forth kind of energy that reminded me of the chess match we played against Miami. After marching down the field, we scored with a 1-yard TD run by Delone Carter. The Pats matched our score when Brady completed a 4-yard pass to Rob Gronkowski for a touchdown. We methodically moved down the field again, and Andrew Luck tossed a 14-yard touchdown pass to T.Y. Hilton.

Brady and the Pats then moved the ball well, but we were able to stop them short of the red zone. Though easily within field goal range, their kicker, Stephen Gostkowski, missed a 36-yard attempt. I was hopeful that this could be our opportunity to take the lead. I couldn't have been more wrong. New England's defense forced us into a three and out, and then Julian Edelman returned our punt for a touchdown, the third one of his career.

Our next possession proved just as disastrous. Aiming for Reggie Wayne, our rookie quarterback threw the ball too high and had it picked off by a new arrival on the Patriots defense, Aqib Talib. Cutting better than many running backs, Talib moved from the right side of the field to the left, eluded the pack of defenders in pursuit, and returned the interception for a touchdown.

Going into halftime we were only behind by a touchdown,

trailing the Patriots 24 – 17. But in the second half our offense coughed up more turnovers, and the defense couldn't hold Brady down. By the end of the game, it was a 59 – 24 rout. After the game, Bruce summed up my thoughts exactly: "We knew we couldn't come in here and turn the football over and have a chance to win. We've got a lot of rookies out there, so every week is a learning experience. This week was a bad learning experience."

We had been so impressed by the great performances of our young players that we forgot they're still rookies. While they had been playing with the maturity and poise of seasoned veterans, these guys still had a lot to learn. We were all humbled by this loss, and it reminded me that my battle wasn't over yet either.

As much as I desperately wanted to trust and believe I would beat cancer, I still had a long way to go. I was tired and still had one chemo treatment left. And even then, there was no guarantee I would be in remission. My mood mirrored the feelings of the players and coaches on the plane returning from Boston. We had made some great advances, but the real fight was just beginning.

U

Chuck, I got your call and text message yesterday. I'm sorry to hear you say you're feeling down. It's easy to fight when we're feeling strong and fresh. But how do we have success in business, success in parenting, and success with our health while overcoming the condition of cancer? We must learn how to fight weary.

I heard a general interviewed on CNN say, "My soldiers in Afghanistan are tired, but they keep fighting." I thought immediately about Gideon. We have to learn how to fight weary, much like Gideon had to do in his victory over the Midianites.

Gideon knew the secret to winning a long, hard battle. Great boxers know it too. They don't just train to knock out their opponent. They are trained to cut the other guy and work the cut. You know all about this. Here's the part you don't know. They are also taught to survive the assault. Some boxers will come out and try to assault their foe and go crazy. When one does, he will box himself out. Chuck, cancer will box itself out if you keep fighting weary and you survive the assault.

Fight weary, my friend. Don't just work the cut, but keep working the cut and survive the assault. Cancer has an assault to it. You survive the assault, and you stay steady. This way you stay even, and people don't even know you are in an assault.

When you start feeling tired and when you feel frustrated, it's a sign you are getting close. Too often people misread the sign and think it means they are far away. "I'm not making progress," they think. But they are. It's the dark before the dawn. You're getting close. Tell yourself when you are tired, "I'm getting close." Survive the assault. The apostle Paul said it best because he knew that if you do not become weary, you will reap in due season if you faint not. That means you're getting close.

I hated to hear you had a couple of bad days, but I love it when you're getting close. As Gideon said, "Fight weary. Keep going." And during the entire time you can barely function, keep whispering to yourself, "Survive the assault."

Elks

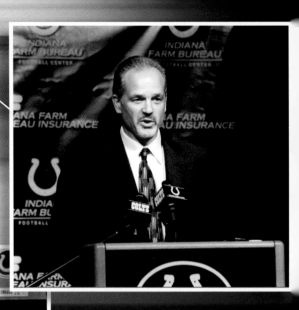

My first press conference as head coach of the Indianapolis Colts, January 26, 2012

Mr. Irsay and I celebrate a win over the Seahawks, October 6, 2013.

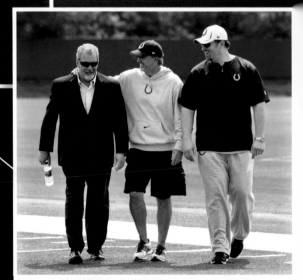

After practice, with Colts owner Mr. Irsay and general manager Ryan Grigson

On the sideline at
Colts-Steelers 2012
preseason game

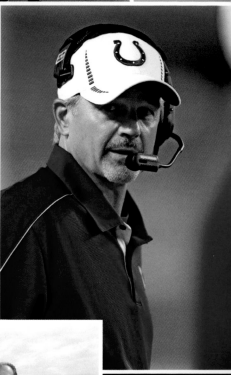

With Ryan and
our first-round
draft pick,
Andrew Luck

2012 preseason game

Family sideline picture with Taylor, Tina , Tori, Tara , Avery, and Addie

My first training camp, with granddaughters Avery and Addie

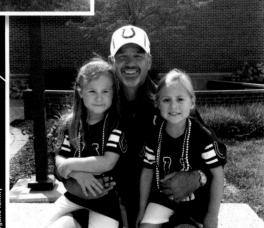

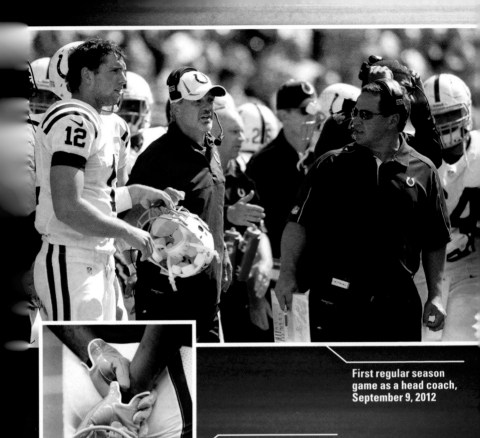

First regular season game as a head coach, September 9, 2012

Reggie Wayne's orange gloves at Green Bay game, October 7, 2012.

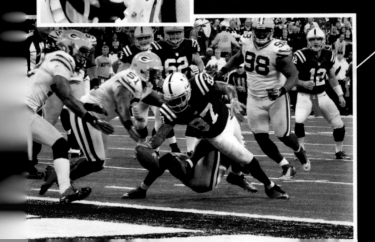

Reggie's gloves in action

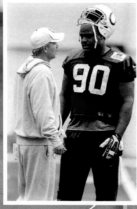

Chatting with Cory Redding at practice

With Antoine Bethea at practice

Sideline

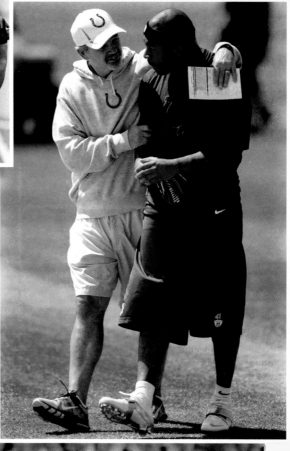

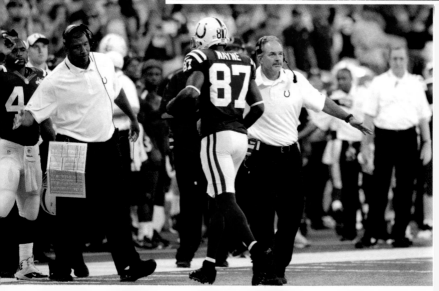

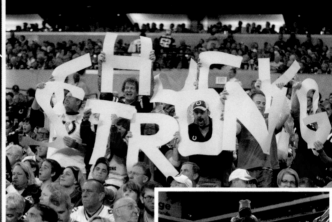

A cheering section at a Colts game lifting up the CHUCK-STRONG cause

© Kevin Terrell/AP Images

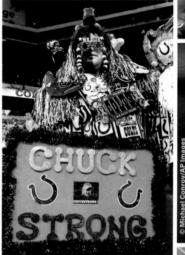

One fan's creative display of support for the CHUCK-STRONG campaign.

© Michael Conroy/AP Images

A get-well card featuring this photo of the entire Colts organization encouraged me during my hospital stay.

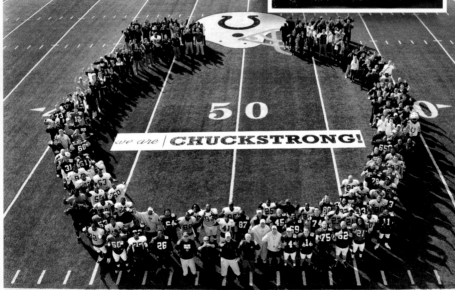

50

we are CHUCKSTRONG!

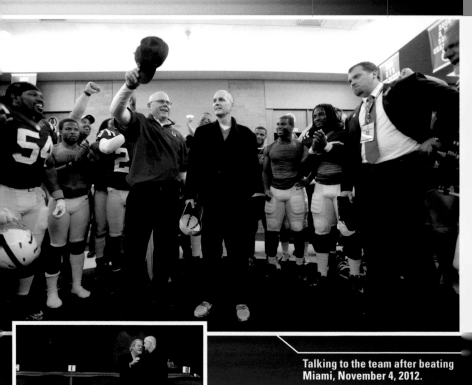

Talking to the team after beating Miami, November 4, 2012.

Enjoying the Colts-Bills game on November 25, 2012, with Mr. Irsay in his stadium suite

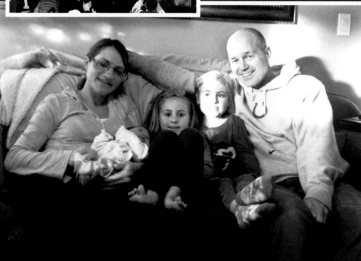

Visiting daughter Tara and grandkids Avery and Addie after Zoey was born

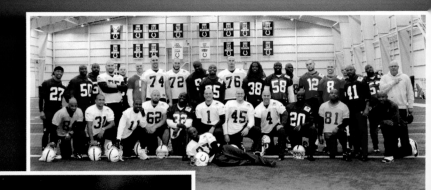

Coin toss

With shaved heads, the Colts show their support

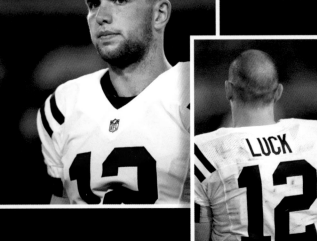

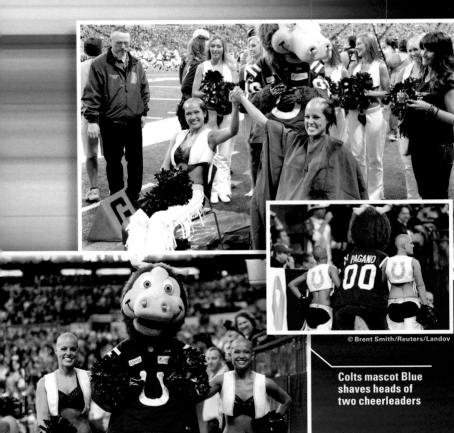

© Brent Smith/Reuters/Landov

Colts mascot Blue shaves heads of two cheerleaders

© Sam Riche/MCT/Landov

© Sam Riche/MCT/Landov

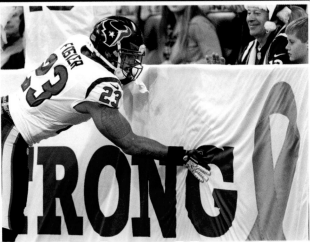

Arian Foster taps banner in support of CHUCKSTRONG

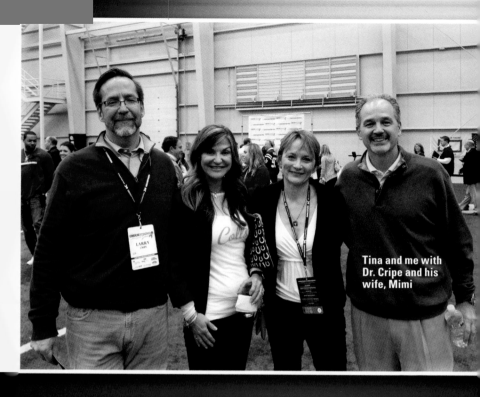

Tina and me with Dr. Cripe and his wife, Mimi

Celebrating Christmas 2012 with Tina in our home

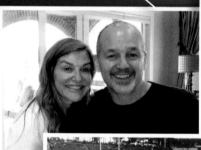

Pagano family

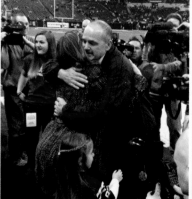

Pagano family

Hugs with my family on the sideline before my first game back as head coach

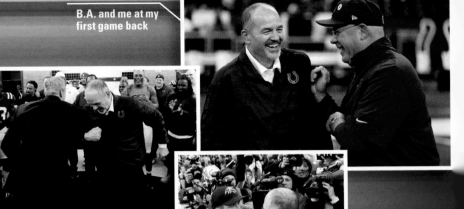

B.A. and me at my first game back

Celebrating with Mr. Irsay after our win over Houston

Postgame chat with Ravens coach John Harbaugh

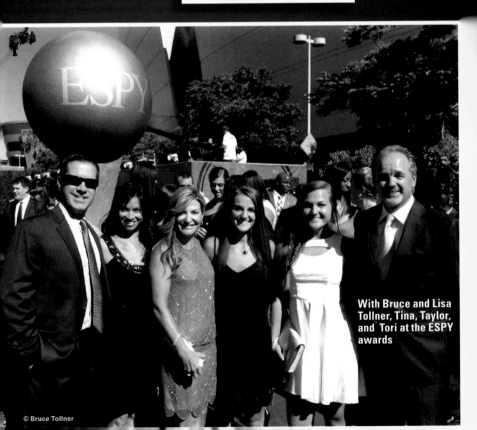

With Bruce and Lisa Tollner, Tina, Taylor, and Tori at the ESPY awards

© Bruce Tollner

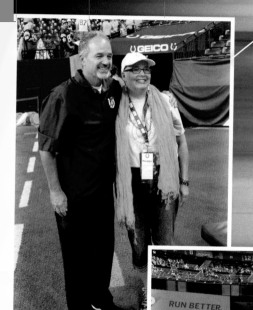

Posing with a fellow cancer survivor before Seahawks game, October 6, 2013

Celebrating cancer victories with a family before 49ers game in San Francisco

My DAD AND Coach PAGANO Beat Cancer

RUN BETTER.

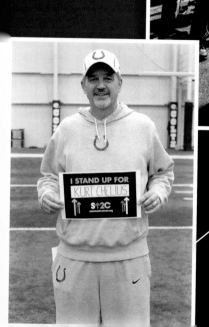

I STAND UP FOR KURT CHELIUS
SU2C
standup2cancer.org

Supporting a fellow cancer fighter

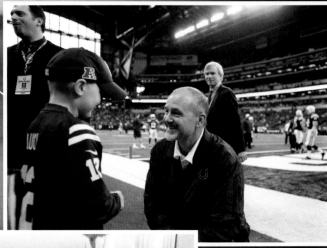

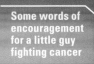
Some words of encouragement for a little guy fighting cancer

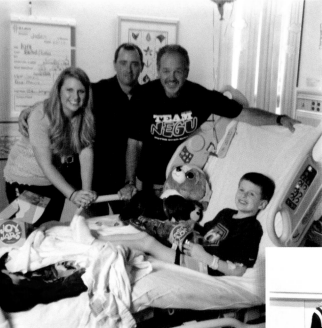

On behalf of the Jessie Rees Foundation, encouraging a courageous child at St. Luke's Children's Hospital in Boise, Idaho, to Never Ever Give Up (NEGU)

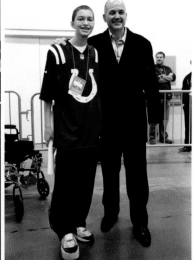

Cory Lane and me before Titans game, December 9, 2012

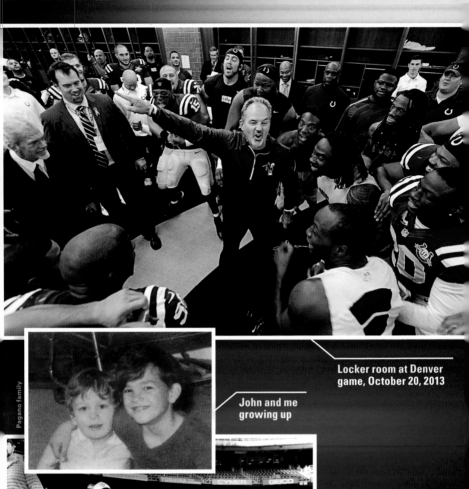

Pagano family

Locker room at Denver
game, October 20, 2013

John and me
growing up

With John and
our parents at
Chargers game
in San Diego,
October 14, 2013

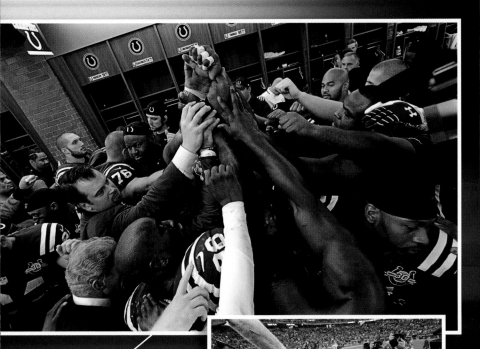

In the locker room at
Broncos game

B.A. and me after Cardinals
game, November 24, 2013

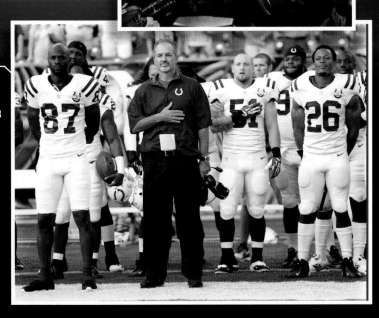

Preseason
game against
the Bengals,
August 29, 2013

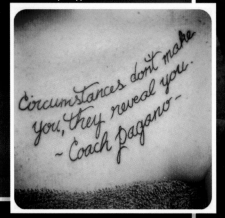
Loyal supporter Jess Schriner

Circumstances don't make you, they reveal you.
~ Coach Pagano ~

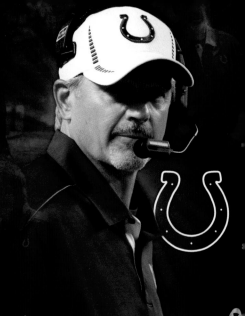

we are | **CHUCKSTRONG**

YOU CAN'T MEASURE
WHAT'S INSIDE A MAN.
YOU CAN'T MEASURE HIS HEART.
AND THESE GUYS GOT MORE
HEART AND GRIT THAN
ANYBODY I'VE EVER
BEEN AROUND.
CHUCK PAGANO

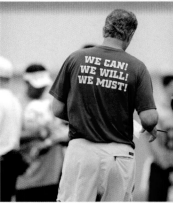

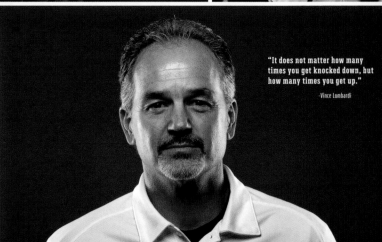

"It does not matter how many
times you get knocked down, but
how many times you get up."

-Vince Lombardi

CHAPTER 9

BALD IS BEAUTIFUL

And Other New Reasons to Celebrate Thanksgiving

As we express our gratitude, we must
never forget that the highest appreciation
is not to utter words, but to live by them.

—John F. Kennedy

Shortly after Thanksgiving, Mr. Irsay surprised Tina and me with an offer to fly us to Boise to see our newest grandchild. Our daughter Tara had just given birth to our third beautiful granddaughter, and we couldn't wait to see her. Because she had been so far along in her pregnancy, Tara had not been able to visit us since I'd gotten sick. So Tina and I were thrilled to accept Mr. Irsay's generous gift to spend a few days with Tara and her husband, Kenny, at their home.

More than ever, we had so much for which to be thankful. I'm a firm believer that Thanksgiving must be a year-round, 365-day celebration and not just a Thursday in November when we eat turkey. Recognizing with gratitude the many blessings in life is critical to keeping a positive attitude. It may sound like a cliché, but it's true. It's a daily attitude of gratitude.

As terrible as it was to be diagnosed with leukemia, I experienced so much love, support, and encouragement from my Colts family, our incredible fans, and all my fellow cancer warriors. And then there was my own family. As we sat around the table with Tara and our grandkids, I got emotional as I thought about all that Tina had done for me. Our relationship had climbed to a new level because of the bond we shared in fighting my cancer together. I don't know how I would've gotten through the past couple of months without her, along with the support from my daughters.

Then to have friends and colleagues like Jim Irsay, Ryan Grigson, Bruce Arians, Pete Ward, and Dan Emerson was simply amazing. Our entire staff and all the assistant coaches. Every one of the players on the football team. There's no way

I can express how much everyone's support meant to me. And most of all, we had reason to give thanks for the great news we had recently received from Dr. Cripe — my cancer was officially *in full remission*. I still had one more round of chemo to complete, but the light at the end of the tunnel was getting brighter.

U

It was so humbling and special for me to see the effort, passion, and creativity that our team was putting into the CHUCK-STRONG campaign. Prior to our second game against the Jags, about three dozen players shaved their heads to show their support for me. Mr. Irsay tweeted, "Buzzed heads and orange locks in honor of Chuck," and when I saw the picture of the guys with their bald heads and big smiles, it made me want to laugh and cry at the same time.

By this time, CHUCKSTRONG had raised over $200,000 for leukemia and cancer research. Some of the guys were doing everything they could think of to raise awareness, motivate fans to contribute, and generate buzz about the cause. Reggie, Andrew, and B.A. partnered with a local restaurant to sign autographs and take pictures with fans to help benefit the Leukemia & Lymphoma Society. Orange stickers showing our Colts horseshoe emblem surrounding my initials had been placed on the nameplates above players' lockers at our team headquarters. Our Colts mascot Blue had donned a Pagano jersey and was sporting orange hair.

Pat McAfee, our punter who had ignited the movement right after I was diagnosed, told a reporter, "Any time you can take a little positive out of a negative experience, I think it's beautiful. That's what CHUCKSTRONG is. We raised so much money — but the only reason is because the man at the head of it is a kick-ass human being. People rallied around Chuck because Chuck Pagano is an amazing dude."

No matter how great Pat's words made me feel, I knew this movement wasn't about me; it was about the human spirit and the will to live, the drive to overcome the odds and beat cancer, not just in my life but for everyone fighting it. CHUCK-STRONG or TINASTRONG or YOURNAMESTRONG is about fighting life's battles, giving it your all, and sticking to it until you win. There were so many other people who were sicker than I was. We all have to stick together and beat this thing. This movement unites us all, because it's rare these days to meet anyone who hasn't had their life touched by cancer, either directly or through their loved ones.

After so many players shaved their heads, I received dozens of pictures of fans who had done the same thing. I'd get a text or open an email, and some stranger would smile back at me with a bald head, telling me they were praying for me, thinking of me and my family, cheering me on, donating money to fight cancer. I cried more than a few times. And it wasn't just guys being so incredibly supportive. As I was about to learn, some very special young women would go to great lengths to show their support as well.

U

I had been cleared to attend our home game that week against Buffalo. While I didn't plan on trying to see everyone in the locker room like I had done before, I couldn't wait to be in the stadium again and see our team in action. I got to visit with a few players before kickoff and then joined Mr. Irsay in his owner's box to watch the game.

The game started with a bang as our rookie receiver T.Y. Hilton returned a punt 75 yards for a touchdown. He was emerging as another breakout player, coming into this matchup with three other games in which his total yards topped 100. I had spoken to him before the game, and based on the practice tapes and game films I'd been watching, I told T.Y. to make "stretch and cut" his new mantra. If he used his strength to propel his body and the ball forward, and his speed to shake defenders and cut into open alleys, I knew he'd break out and score some touchdowns.

T.Y. gave us a bit of a scare, though, on his second punt return. He got sandwiched in a high-low hit combination that left him motionless on the ground for several minutes. You never want to see a player lying motionless like that after a play. I felt like I was holding my breath until he got on his feet and walked off the field. He was taken to the locker room to be examined for a possible head injury or concussion. I said a prayer, hoping for the best, as the first half ended with us leading 13 – 6.

I had heard something really special was scheduled for halftime, and I can't convey just how amazing it was. Apparently, earlier in the week our mascot Blue had tweeted out a CHUCKSTRONG challenge: If he could raise $10,000 by game time, he was challenging any Colts cheerleader to step forward and get her head shaved. It was a crazy stunt, and being the father of three daughters, I know how women feel about their hair. Not one but *two* of our cheerleaders, Megan and Crystal Anne, accepted Blue's challenge. As a result, CHUCKSTRONG raised $22,000 to benefit leukemia research at the Simon Cancer Center — and the women were about to get their haircuts at halftime.

With the promise that they'd donate their beautiful, brunette, shoulder-length hair to Locks of Love, a nonprofit organization that provides wigs and hairpieces to children suffering hair loss related to their medical conditions, Megan and Crystal Anne smiled and held hands as Blue pulled the barber shears across their heads. The crowd went wild!

These young women looked truly radiant — far better than I did with no hair. Interviewed after the game, Megan responded to the thank-yous she received in such a humble, classy way. "I just shaved my head. But these people are going through the battle for their lives — they're really the ones who deserve all the praise," she said.

It was simply amazing. As we pulled ahead to win the game, in the fourth quarter I stepped out of the owner's box with Mr. Irsay and waved to the crowd. As the cameras zoomed in on me, everyone in the stadium was soon on their feet. Over 64,000 people were clapping, cheering, and chanting, "Chuck! Strong! Chuck! Strong!" Tears formed in my eyes, and words completely escaped me. So I patted my heart several times and simply mouthed, "Thank you."

The players achieved their goal by beating the Bills 20 – 13. Bruce had told them before the game that I was going to be there watching. "We want him leaving this place with a huge smile on his face!" he told them. As I left Lucas Oil Stadium that Sunday afternoon, I couldn't quit smiling.

U

By the beginning of December, when most people are thinking of the holidays, doing their Christmas shopping, and planning their office parties and family dinners, football teams begin looking ahead at playoff scenarios. We were in the hunt.

Several sports commentators thought we had the inside track for the AFC wild-card spot, but our team knew we couldn't assume we'd make it or take anything for granted. After such a memorable, emotional home game, we now had to face a tough opponent, the Detroit Lions, on the road.

The Lions gave us a heck of a game. Going against the league's leading receiver, Calvin Johnson (nicknamed "Megatron" after one of the Transformers because of his size and large hands), and a young quarterback with a great arm, Matthew Stafford, we knew it could be an explosive, high-scoring game — and it was. In the end, it came down to the last 4 seconds of the game. Even though we'd played a great game, we trailed 33 – 28 with time running out.

Facing fourth down with those precious 4 seconds left on the clock, Andrew took a calculated risk that receiver Donnie Avery could get open and make it to the end zone — and he did. Catching the short pass, Avery ran 14 yards, untouched, to score the winning touchdown with no time left on the clock.

Afterward, Bruce Arians told an interviewer, "Some teams find ways to win in clutch situations, and others don't." From my experience, the key was never to give up, just to keep giving your all on every single play — even the last one. Which is exactly what our guys did to defeat the Lions. Now our record had improved to 9 – 4, and we were guaranteed to win more than half of our regular season games.

In December it's tough not to think about the playoffs, which only intensified my impatience to get back on the sideline with our team. We were all looking ahead, working hard to play games beyond the regular season, but I wanted life to return to normal, to be back doing my job. Although I had just finished chemo, I needed to regain my strength before returning to work. And our team had to keep winning and finish the season. All the more reason to just focus on one game at a time, one play at a time, one day at a time.

It was that easy. And it was that hard.

U

After such a dramatic comeback win, our team morale was off the charts. The guys heard I would likely be coming back for our last game of the season, and they were determined to carry us into postseason play. For the third time since being diagnosed with leukemia, I would be attending the next game at home, against the Tennessee Titans. We had squeezed out a win against them in overtime back in October, but this time I was worried they had our number.

We were riding such an emotional high as the CHUCK-STRONG campaign kept gaining momentum and press coverage and, best of all, passed the quarter-million-dollar mark in contributions to fight cancer. I was in constant contact with players and coaches, as well as with Mr. Irsay and Ryan, and their only concern was that I not overdo it and put stress on my weak immune system. They knew how badly I wanted to be back, but they also wanted me back for more than just one game or even for just this season. They knew I wanted to be coaching the Colts for the rest of my career.

It's funny, too, but every now and then a reporter or friend outside the Colts' organization would ask me if I was worried about losing my job since Bruce was doing such a great job. It never crossed my mind — for at least two big reasons. First and foremost, I trusted Mr. Irsay implicitly and knew without a doubt that his integrity, loyalty, and support never wavered.

The second major reason emerges from my trust of Bruce Arians. Hiring him as our offensive coordinator was truly a godsend. In addition to carrying out all the normal responsibilities of being a head coach, Bruce had added a layer — staying in constant communication with me, encouraging me, answering my questions about individual plays and players, and just being my friend. No matter how entrenched B.A. was in his daily duties as head coach in my absence, first and foremost on his mind was the fact that his friend was fighting cancer. Both Mr. Irsay and Bruce made it clear I had job security.

U

If I didn't have a heart condition before the 2012 season, it sure felt like I might have one before it was over. We had pulled out so many close games that it was unbelievable. Andrew continued to exceed our expectations. He now was tied with two-time Super Bowl champion Ben Roethlisberger and Vince Young for being a rookie quarterback with five fourth-quarter comebacks. And our next game would give him a chance to try to break that tie.

The first half against Tennessee definitely didn't go our way. In fact, it was disastrous. As he was being pulled to the ground by a defender intent on the sack, Andrew made an uncharacteristic decision to throw the ball. The Titans' Will Witherspoon grabbed an easy pick-six to give his team a two-score lead. With a 31-yard field goal added in the last seconds before halftime, Tennessee led 20 – 7.

Opening the third quarter, the offense moved down the field on a methodical 80-yard drive that culminated in a 1-yard touchdown run by Delone Carter. I think the real turning point occurred, however, when Pat McAfee punted the ball 52 yards and out of bounds at Tennessee's 1-yard line. After Cassius Vaughn intercepted a bad throw by the Titans' quarterback and ran 3 easy yards for a touchdown, we led 21 – 20 late in the third quarter. In the last quarter of the game, both teams added field goals, our two to their one, and we ran out the clock for yet another amazing come-from-behind win. Final score, Colts 27, Titans 23.

Later that day we found out that division rivals Cincinnati and Pittsburgh both lost their games. Suddenly, the math was simple. We were one win away from heading to the playoffs. One win.

∪

Good morning, Chuck. Back in 2007, our mutual friend Butch Davis called me right after his dentist discovered a cancerous growth in his mouth that was diagnosed as non-Hodgkin lymphoma. I told Butch I had worked at a cancer support center in Pittsburgh, and from that experience, I became convinced that so many of the patients who survive cancer are those who are most determined to beat it. The question is, How bad do you want it?

What I have observed is that the disease and its treatment wear people down. Sure, it's easy for me to say, "You've got to want to beat it." But I know that when you've been sick with cancer for one month, two months, three in a row from the chemotherapy treatments, it takes all the fight out of you. But like so many things in life, it's a matter of how badly we want something, and what we are willing to do to get what we want.

Chuck, our enemy's tool is often fatigue. Often it's not some big temptation that derails our faith as much as the weariness from just trying to hang on. Do you want to serve God more than you want to allow that fatigue to wear you out? Do you want to stand on the sideline and coach your team? Do you want to tell your story to people so you can inspire them to overcome adversity? Do you want to make a difference in people's lives? Do you want to show others how to rise higher? How bad do you want it?

In 1970 Stanford University professors conducted a study at the Bing Nursery School on the campus. The purpose of this study, which became known as the marshmallow test, was to understand the control of deferred gratification, and more than six hundred children participated in the experiment. Children were placed in a room where there were no distractions, except for a treat of their choice — a marshmallow, cookie, or pretzel — placed on a table. The children could eat the snack right away; however, if they waited fifteen minutes without giving in to the immediate urge, they would be rewarded with two snacks. Some children ate the marshmallow immediately; others delayed for five or six minutes. Only one-third were able to earn the reward. The researchers followed the participants for twenty-five years, and the ones who had the discipline to resist eating the marshmallow became the most successful in life. Not surprisingly, the ones with the least willpower were the least successful.

Chuck, don't eat the marshmallow. How bad do you want to beat this thing? How bad do you want to win? Paul said that if we do not grow weary, we will reap in due season, as long as we don't faint. Fight the good fight — you're almost there!

Elks

CHAPTER 10

FINISHING STRONG

Back on the Sideline and Headed to the Playoffs

A dream doesn't become reality through magic;
it takes sweat, determination and hard work.

—Colin Powell

When we're kids, Christmas is all about waiting for Santa, getting together with cousins and extended family, opening presents, and playing with new toys. As adults, we often enjoy recapturing those special memories by experiencing the true meaning of Christmas, the celebration of the birth of Christ — a time of joy and peace, of giving back to those people in our lives who give so much. As December 25, 2012, approached, I knew that no matter how we celebrated, it would be a Christmas unlike any other.

Because I grew up in Colorado, we had many white Christmases, and I can remember holiday snowball fights and afternoons spent sledding or skiing. For as long as I can recall, football has always been a part of Christmas for me as well. Growing up, I watched my dad coach end-of-season and championship games and later played in them myself before becoming a coach. Between the many college bowl games and the race for the NFL playoffs, it wouldn't be Christmas in the Pagano house without football.

This year was no different. With three regular season games left, we needed to win at least one of them to clinch the AFC wild-card spot in the playoffs. We had come so far — all of us. As an organization committed to excellence, the Colts had already overcome the prior season's struggles to return to its high standards of success. As a young team with a rookie quarterback, other rookies in key roles, new players, and a rookie absentee coach, the 2012 Colts consistently dug deep and found ways to win games they weren't supposed to be able to win. As a middle-aged man diagnosed with leukemia only three months prior, I wasn't supposed to be back on my feet, regaining my strength and beating the odds the way I was now.

The reason that all three of us — the organization, this year's team, and myself — had come so far boils down to this one thing: We refused to allow anyone else to tell us what we could and could not do. We purposed in our hearts that no one else would be allowed to write our story's next chapter for us. We would find the grit, the determination, and the strength to move through adversity and win.

To this point in the season, we had not lost two games in a row. When we made mistakes, we owned them and learned from them. When we failed on one play, we shook it off and stayed focused on the next. When I didn't feel like getting out of bed on those mornings I was having chemo treatments, I did it anyway. There simply was no other choice. I had a loving wife and children counting on me to be there for them, and I loved them too much to stop trying. I also desperately wanted to get back to coaching football.

I know it's not easy. It never is. If winning were easy, it wouldn't be worth it. I also know that so many other people had it much harder than I did — facing other types of cancer, not responding to treatment the way I did, or not having the incredible medical attention and personal support that I was blessed to receive. But regardless of our circumstances, they do not define us — not unless we give in and let them. Circumstances never determine who we are; they reveal who we are.

U

Having completed my last chemo treatment in early December, I truly felt like a kid at Christmas. I felt stronger each week, and the best medicine I received came from our team. Intent on returning for that last game of the season — as well as on coaching every game we played in the postseason — I stayed connected to everyone on the team like never before. I'm sure they thought I was going overboard at times, but if they did, they never showed it or complained about it.

After our win over the Titans, we headed to Houston for a division matchup against the Texans who had just been stung by a loss to New England in a tough game similar to our own against the Pats. They were eager to make up for their performance the week before by beating us to clinch the AFC South title. We had won three consecutive games, taking our record to 9 – 4, and the title would belong to us if we could beat Houston.

I was especially concerned because we were missing two key offensive linemen because of injuries — center Samson Satele and right tackle Winston Justice — and Houston had an outstanding defense featuring J.J. Watt, who led the AFC in total number of sacks. Having grown up in the Houston area, Andrew Luck was eager to put on a great performance in his hometown.

He ended up being sacked a total of five times, three at the hands of Watt. We couldn't contain the Texans' offense the way we wanted to either. By halftime, we trailed 20 – 3. But we had come from behind to win with larger deficits before. Late in the third quarter, we were finally back in the game, breathing down their necks and within six points of the lead. But then we began to fall apart, as Houston held on to win.

They used their great running back Arian Foster to chew up time on the clock, keeping us from getting the ball. Foster ran for a season-high 165 yards, taking him over 1,300 yards for the season. And when we did get the ball, their defense kept us from finding our groove. We ended up drawing an unsportsmanlike conduct penalty and were forced to punt the ball. Bruce knew we were so close, and yet we just couldn't seem to find our rhythm in this game. After the game he told reporters, "It was a tough loss for us in that we came here with one idea, and that was to win the division. And we're not going to win the division — they did."

∪

Along with the rest of the team, I refused to entertain any possibility we would not win another game and not go to the playoffs to enter my mind. We would win one, if not both, of our remaining games and secure that wild-card slot on the road to the Super Bowl. Facing the Kansas City Chiefs at Arrowhead Stadium, never an easy place to win, we knew we had to come together as a team intent on nothing short of winning.

We jumped out to an early lead when Darius Butler intercepted a pass on the Chiefs' fifth play of their opening drive and returned it 32 yards for a touchdown. We added a couple of field goals by Adam Vinatieri, while they only managed one field goal, taking us into halftime with a 13 – 3 lead.

On the first play of the third quarter, though, the Chiefs clawed their way back. Jamaal Charles cut left, found an open alley along the sideline, and then cut to the middle of the field, winning a foot race against our defenders in hot pursuit. His 86-yard touchdown made it a 3-point game. Later in the third quarter, the Chiefs missed a chance to take the lead when Brady Quinn's pass was picked off by Vontae Davis in the end zone. They held us to a three and out and then managed to make a field goal to tie the game.

Although Andrew Luck had broken Cam Newton's NFL record for total passing yards in a season by a rookie quarterback in the second quarter of this game, our offense struggled in the third quarter. In fact, Andrew went through a rough stretch and went 1 for 13. What I love about Andrew, though, is his patience and persistence. As I've said before, he does a great job of having amnesia — one of the best traits a quarterback can have. He remains calm, poised, and determined, and he keeps playing the game, one play at a time.

Our defense stepped up too. When the Chief's Brady Quinn tried a quarterback sneak on fourth and inches, our defense stuffed him, giving us the ball and setting the stage for another fourth-quarter, come-from-behind win. Faced with third down, Andrew hit T.Y. Hilton for an 11-yard completion that set up another series of downs, including yet another crucial third-down play. In the clutch once again, Andrew came through with a 7-yard touchdown strike to Reggie Wayne in the end zone. We had become the comeback kings, with a total of seven games this season in which we'd pulled out a win in the fourth quarter or in overtime.

"At times it looked a little bleak," Bruce Arians explained after the game. "But our guys hung in there and made plays when they had to make them. Offensively we struggled and then put together a drive, just like we have all year." With our record now at 10 – 5, we became only the second team (the other being the Dolphins in 2008) to win 10 games after losing 14 or more games the previous season.

We had secured the AFC wild-card spot.

We were going to the playoffs.

∪

The day after our victory over the Chiefs, I returned to work for the first time in three months. The light was still on in my office, just as Bruce had left it while I was gone. There's no other way to describe it — it was like coming home again. In terms of outcomes, this final regular season game meant next to nothing in terms of the playoff picture. But it meant everything to me.

In one of those scheduling flukes that seem to happen late in a season, we once again faced our opponents from two weeks ago, the Houston Texans. Only this time, there were two huge differences. The first was that we would be playing at home, our last game in what had been a strange, unexpected, and miraculous season. The second was that I would be there — not watching on TV from the hospital, not watching from home, not even watching from the stadium box with Ryan and Tom Telesco. I would be back on the sideline again.

The last few months had been such an emotional time, so many ups and downs and back and forths, three steps forward and two steps back. So much of my journey with leukemia had paralleled those come-from-behind games we had become so good at winning. It's easy to compare life to a football game, but the qualities needed to win in both never seemed clearer to me. Who you are off the field is who you are on the field. How you face each day, every day, is how you handle play after play of each game.

When I accepted Mr. Irsay's offer to become the head coach of the Indianapolis Colts, I had no idea my life would become so inextricably interwoven with the lives of everyone in this organization. I had no idea that cancer was growing in my body and would require me to miss three-quarters of my first regular season in my new role. And I had no idea just how much I would come to depend on the support, encouragement, and friendship of my new family.

Walking onto the field for our last game of the season was like walking onto a football field for the first time again. It was like being a kid again, waking up on Christmas morning and opening the best present ever, the one you'd been wanting for a long time.

U

Despite the incredible joy and excitement, I also felt really nervous being back on the field. I knew everyone would be watching me, reading my body language to see how I was feeling both physically and emotionally. And as much as I loved and appreciated everyone's support, I didn't want to be a distraction from the game. We were there to play the last game of the season, and that's all I wanted to do.

But I'd be lying if I didn't tell you how great it also felt to be back there. Walking onto the field, my family on the sideline. I had never experienced such an overwhelming sense of support from everyone. We waved to fans, and that's when the stadium's two Jumbotrons began playing a tribute video, tracing my journey this season and describing the phenomenal success that CHUCKSTRONG had accomplished in the fight against cancer. It was emotional for all of us.

Andrew Luck and our offense worked methodically downfield, covering 75 yards in 13 plays and chewing up over 7 minutes on the clock. Coby Fleener caught a 1-yard touchdown pass, and we were off and running. The Texans tried to get something going, but then Vontae Davis picked off Houston quarterback Matt Schaub's deep pass and returned it 26 yards. With the ball back in our possession, Andrew connected with

T.Y. Hilton on a key pass, setting up Vick Ballard's touchdown from the 1-yard line right before halftime.

I didn't envy Houston having to play us in such an emotionally charged environment. Unlike us, their seed placement for the playoffs would be hurt if they lost this game. Motivated by the prospect of home-field advantage in the postseason if they beat us, Houston took the lead in the third quarter when premier running back Arian Foster broke through a bottleneck and ran 13 yards for a touchdown. But it's what he did after he scored that I'll never forget. Arian dashed through the end zone and affectionately patted the CHUCKSTRONG banner before bowing in front of it. Classy move by a classy man.

Shortly after Foster's score, the Texans, trailing by only one point, got the ball back again. We held them to a field goal, but they were in the lead late in the third quarter.

On the kickoff return, Deji Karim caught the ball in the end zone and ran it out. Like a bullet train flying off the tracks, he zipped through a seam down the middle and never looked back. No one touched him for almost 80 yards, and he completed his 101-yard return in the opposite end zone from which he started. I raced along the sideline, along with the rest of the staff and players. Later, I would find out Karim's runback was the longest return since the Colts moved to Indy in 1984.

The celebration continued into the fourth quarter. Faced with a third and 23 on our own 30-yard line, Andrew hit T.Y. with a perfectly thrown missile, which he took to the house for a touchdown. We went on to win the game, 28 – 16.

What a way to come home!

U

After we won, we all started hugging and high-fiving. It was an awesome feeling. I was surrounded by our players, assistant coaches, staff — even the Texans, as head coach Gary Kubiak and many of his players congratulated me warmly. Fans and reporters were milling around on the field, and it was truly an incredible celebration, a fitting end to one of the wildest, most spectacular football seasons ever.

In the locker room, the party continued. Hugs, high fives, laughter, and dancing continued. Mr. Irsay presented me with the game ball, and, once again, words can't describe just how grateful and overjoyed I felt at that moment. Players started cheering and playing music, and Mr. Irsay and I joined in the victory dance. I just kept telling all of them, "Thank you" and "Love you" over and over again.

As I sat in front of the cameras at the postgame press conference, I was tired but elated. "What a day, what a day!" I said smiling to the crowded room of reporters. I told them how we could easily talk about the game we'd just played and all the amazing players and plays that occurred, many for the record books. But I also made it clear that what we had just seen out there was something I'd been watching for the past twelve weeks.

I explained what a dream come true this game was for me and compared my return to coaching like getting on a bike again and having it all come back. You just jump back on and start pedaling. This was where I was meant to be, doing what I was meant to be doing. I concluded by telling reporters how proud I was of these guys for doing what we all had just done together.

"We refuse to live in circumstances," I said. "We live in vision."

U

Hey, Chuck—Elks here. When I was in my junior year in college, majoring in the unlikely combination of biology and coaching, I was in the library and came across a book on sports psychology. I was so intrigued by it that I spent the entire afternoon reading it. An unusual combination, but it fascinated me.

Ten years later, I had my doctorate and was presenting a paper at the University of West Virginia. Only three people were present, and when I finished, they all walked out without saying a word to me. I thought I had bombed. Eight months later, I walked into my office at the university, and the secretary said, "You just got an invitation to work with the United States Olympic Committee. Call this number if you're interested."

"What?" I said.

"When you presented that paper last April, one of those men was the vice president of the Olympic Committee. He wants you to call him."

It was a dream come true. I became an intern in Colorado Springs working with athletes who would represent the United States at the 1988 Olympics in the summer in Seoul, Korea, and the winter in Calgary, Alberta, Canada.

It's amazing how all of this worked out for me. You say things; you think things—and sure enough, things happen. Viktor Frankl wrote a paper titled "Gymnasium" in 1923 on the psychology of philosophical thinking. He studied medicine at the University of Vienna and later specialized in neurology and psychiatry.

A Jew, Frankl was deported to the Auschwitz concentration camp in October 1944, and then to Dachau until his liberation by the Americans in April 1945. Throughout his horrific imprison-ment and subsequent brutal treatment at the hands of the Nazis, Frankl contemplated the meaning of life. Even in his misery, he concluded that the striving to find meaning in one's life is the primary and most powerful motivating force in humans. Years later, this theory became the basis of logotherapy, which he wrote about in his famous book, Man's Search for Meaning.

Chuck, there is a lot to be said about thinking about something and then seeing it happen. Your dreams are coming true, so keep visualizing them every day. I want you to have four dif-ferent scripts. Write them out in detail. Like a dream, visualize coaching on the sideline, and see yourself as healthy as can be. See yourself running up and down the sideline. You're hugging players, screaming at B.A. because he called a bad play. You're thrilled about what's going on. You're high-fiving the guys. The Colts are pulling out another comeback victory.

Also put in your script that you and Tina are in Florence. No kids or grandkids with you — just you and Tina. Then the two of you are in Naples. You're eating wonderful meals, drinking good wine. Again, you're as healthy as can be and having the time of your lives. You're celebrating your love and being together through everything.

Let's now do a third script. This time you see yourself walking down the aisle with your daughter. She is wearing a white gown and looks beautiful. You are both emotional. Tina is waiting down there for you. The priest asks, "Who gives this young lady?" Feel the emotion. Then I want you to see yourself dancing at the reception.

Okay, Chuck, now for the last one. I want you to see yourself winning the Super Bowl. Picture yourself getting that Lombardi Trophy. You're hoisting it up, and the crowd is roaring!

I miss you, and I'm going to come out and see you soon. We're going to celebrate all the great things in your life — both now and to come. That's what I am visualizing right now!

CHAPTER 11

AFC WILD-CARD GAME

Losing the Game and Winning the Team

Endurance is not just the ability to bear
a hard thing, but to turn it into glory.

—William Barclay

I n football, you can never go home again.

We would be returning to Baltimore to face my former team, the Ravens, in the AFC wild-card game. I say returning because, as most football fans know, the Colts originated in Baltimore. Despite the three decades that have passed since the franchise moved to Indianapolis, the circumstances of that historic transition remain controversial. Maybe a little history of the club would be helpful.

A group of fans and investors brought a franchise to Baltimore in the early 1950s, and the team was named the Colts. The name honored Baltimore's long history of horse racing, including its historic tradition of hosting the annual Preakness, part of that sport's Triple Crown. That original franchise was dissolved within a year, as the sport of professional football experienced growing pains during the formation of what would eventually become the National Football League.

In 1953, businessman Carroll Rosenbloom brought an NFL franchise back to Baltimore, and a naming contest by fans restored the Colts name. Led by legendary quarterback Johnny Unitas, the team won championships in 1958 and 1959. In Super Bowl III, the Colts were upset by the New York Jets after a record-breaking winning season, but in 1970 they returned to win Super Bowl V against the Dallas Cowboys.

In 1972, Rosenbloom traded the franchise to another businessman, Robert Irsay, the father of our current owner, Jim Irsay. Robert had bid successfully on purchasing the Los Angeles Rams from the estate of its deceased owner and then immediately negotiated a deal to swap franchises with Rosenbloom.

The Colts enjoyed successful seasons in the mid-1970s, winning three division titles but losing in each of the playoffs. Then in the late '70s and early '80s, the team went through a dramatic slump of losing seasons, and fan attendance declined. During this period, Robert Irsay discussed plans for a new stadium with both city of Baltimore and state of Maryland officials. An agreement could not be reached, however, and it became clear that the frustrated owner would likely move the team to another city. Several — including Memphis, Jacksonville, New York, Indianapolis, and Phoenix — had openly courted him for months, even years.

At an impasse in negotiations and fearful the Colts would move, Baltimore city officials in March 1984 persuaded state lawmakers to take dramatic steps and to attempt obtaining the franchise by eminent domain. At that point, Robert Irsay, with the help of government leaders in Indiana, loaded up trucks and moved the team overnight to Indianapolis. Despite legal proceedings from the city of Baltimore, the courts upheld the move. But lifelong Baltimore Colts fans have not been quite as forgiving, despite the fact that a new franchise, the Baltimore Ravens, brought football back to the city in 1996.

Now we were preparing to take the Indianapolis Colts back to Baltimore to play the Ravens in the AFC wild-card game. Because of my four-year coaching stint in Baltimore, my family and I had many close ties to the current Ravens football team, as well as to the area.

Returning for this game would be bittersweet in many ways. While Tina and I looked forward to a reunion with friends and former colleagues in Baltimore, our hearts and our home were now in the Midwest. The incredibly generous, supporting, and loving Colts we knew hailed from Indianapolis.

Like I said, in football, sometimes it's tough to go home again.

U

I knew firsthand that our game against the Ravens would be a tough one. After spending four years there, I could testify to the strength of the team, the passion of its fans, and the leadership of head coach John Harbaugh. Baltimore had a top-notch organization, and they were hungry to win.

Like many specialized fields, professional football is a small world, and you know eventually you may end up playing against someone you once coached with, as well as against players you once coached. As it turned out, not only would I be playing my old team, but my predecessor as head coach of the Indianapolis Colts, Jim Caldwell, was now the Ravens' offensive coordinator.

While our team had rallied together and played for a cause bigger than just winning, it was clear the Ravens would also be playing with a passionate purpose as well. On Wednesday prior to the game, Ray Lewis announced he would be retiring after the postseason. He had missed most of the regular season with a torn triceps muscle but had healed enough to play again, at least in a few games.

Ray is a phenomenal player, a gifted linebacker, and we shared ties going back to the University of Miami, where he played his college ball. Drafted by the Ravens in their inaugural season, Ray had earned numerous awards and frequent trips to the Pro Bowl. After playing seventeen seasons, all for the Ravens, this future first-ballot Hall of Famer had decided to retire.

I coached Ray directly during my time in Baltimore and knew the level of intensity he brings to the game when he's on the field. Anyone who's been fortunate enough to spend time around him knows what an incredible man, leader, and athlete he is. I knew Ray Lewis would not be retiring without a fight on the field. I knew his team would do everything in their power to send him out in style — with a Super Bowl ring.

∪

My chemo was now over, and my cancer was in remission — and I had a family, friends, and a team that had supported me. The fact that our team was now playing in the AFC wild-card game only added to my happiness. Yet, as much as I love football, I knew it was just a game on the field, not the life-or-death battle I had witnessed in the eyes of so many brave boys and girls, men and women fighting cancer.

Other than visiting with patients on my floor at the Simon Cancer Center, I had many other opportunities to meet cancer patients and cancer survivors. After I returned home and began attending games again, I met several kids from Riley Hospital who had been sponsored by CHUCKSTRONG and invited to a game. They got to meet players, sit in special seats, and go out on the field for the coin toss.

At our home game against Buffalo on November 25, 2012, when our two cheerleaders shaved their heads, some of the kids there with cancer had shaved theirs too. A young girl named Mickey Deputy wanted to shave her head in support of CHUCKSTRONG. I got to meet her in the tunnel just before the game started, just before she and some other kids went out onto the field for the coin toss. She was such a joy — so excited to be a part of our team and to know we were all in the same fight together. No one who has cancer is alone in their battle.

I also got to meet a special young man named Cory Lane. Cory got out of his wheelchair and gave me a big hug and said, "Hey, Coach, you can beat this thing. You're tough enough." His words mean so much to me even now, because I know he spoke for all of us.

I stayed in touch with many of those kids through letters and emails. It wasn't long after I met Cory when he lost his battle with cancer. My heart breaks when I think about him and all the millions of lives taken by cancer. Our war on cancer is not over. It will never end until there's a cure for kids like Cory Lane.

"Hey, Coach, you can beat this thing. You're tough enough."

U

Bruce got sick and missed a couple of practices that week. Feeling better, he joined us for our pregame meal, only to have his symptoms return. Our team doctors checked him out and called an ambulance to take him to the hospital. After he had gone through some tests, we learned he'd be fine but would have to miss the game.

As disappointed as we all were, after what we had been through together, it was next man up. Clyde Christensen, our quarterbacks coach, would be calling the plays in Bruce's place.

The game itself was, in fact, the struggle I had expected. As excited as we were to be there, our game play in Baltimore lacked our usual intensity and focus. It wasn't just us; the Ravens couldn't seem to find their rhythm either. Early in the game, running back Ray Rice fumbled and Ray Lewis dropped what looked like an easy interception. Not that we weren't grateful. We had plenty of our own frustrations, including a fumble by Andrew Luck after he was sacked and stripped of the ball.

After a scoreless first quarter, Baltimore finally scored. Rice netted a 47-yard gain on a screen pass from quarterback Joe Flacco, which led to a 2-yard touchdown run by Vonta Leach. We followed with two long field goals from Adam Vinatieri, a 47-yarder and a 52-yarder, and the Ravens added one of their own, propelling them into halftime with a 10 – 6 lead.

During the second half, we never got our offense going. Ray Lewis clearly had our number and kept the Ravens' defense fired up against us. We added another field goal in the third quarter but wouldn't score again. Flacco connected with Dennis Pitta for a 20-yard touchdown in the same period. But it was receiver Anquan Boldin who had the big day. With five catches for 145 yards, Bolden caught the last one in the fourth quarter for a touchdown, sealing our loss, with the final score being 24 – 9.

The Baltimore Ravens would go on to win Super Bowl XLVII against the San Francisco 49ers.

U

While it's always disappointing to lose, it was hard to complain after the incredible turnaround we'd experienced during that 2012 season. September seemed a lifetime ago. I was just getting my strength back, and now our season and postseason were over.

I had nothing to regret or feel down about, though. We laid a strong foundation for the next year's team and had seen so many talented but inexperienced players step up and improve over the season. Our selection of Andrew Luck clearly had been the right one. Time and time again, he played like a veteran of several years and not a young man in his first NFL season. We found our franchise quarterback for many years to come.

The unity we experienced by overcoming adversity together was priceless. You can't buy the kind of brotherhood we had with one another over the course of those previous four months. And now we were able to celebrate together — not only my return and a winning season, but also the bittersweet news we received from Bruce. He had been asked to become the head coach for the Arizona Cardinals and accepted the position on January 17, 2013. As much as I hated to see him leave the Colts, I was thrilled for my old friend who had been like a brother to me during those past months.

He had pretty much resigned himself to retiring without ever being a head coach in the NFL. Then the onset of my leukemia thrust Bruce into the role of interim head coach. I knew he was more than up to the challenge. Bruce is a great coach and teacher, and now he finally had the opportunity to lead an organization.

In February 2013, Bruce was voted AP's Coach of the Year, an award never before given to an interim coach. He had led the Colts to a 9 – 3 record during the twelve weeks I was away. Almost a year prior, we had hired him to run the Colts' offense, and neither of us could have ever imagined the wild turn of events that now led to his departure. But I was truly happy for Bruce — he more than deserved the accolades, the recognition, and the position of head coach with the Cardinals. He's a good man and even when I have to face him on the opposite side of the field, he will always be like family to me.

U

We had come so far in such a short amount of time. The 2012 Indianapolis Colts team achieved many records and milestones, secondary to what we achieved as a unified team but significant nonetheless. Our team became only the second team in NFL history to rebound by winning ten or more games in a season after losing fourteen or more the previous season. The Miami Dolphins in 2008 were the only other team to achieve the same turnaround.

First-round draft pick and rookie quarterback Andrew Luck finished the season with the NFL record for passing yards by a rookie and broke the team record for most completions in a season. He won 11 games, the most by a rookie quarterback taken as the No. 1 pick in the draft — and also the most wins in Colts history by a rookie QB. He led seven game-winning drives in the fourth quarter or in overtime, tying league records. Andrew set NFL rookie records with 4,374 yards passing and 627 attempts. He also notched a team record with his five rushing touchdowns.

Reggie Wayne finished the season ranked tenth in NFL history for number of receptions — 968. He moved up to No. 14 all-time with 13,063 yards. He also set an NFL record with at least three catches in 64 consecutive games. Reggie led our team in receiving yards for a sixth straight season and tied Marvin Harrison's team record for number of receptions, also breaking Harrison's record for leading the team in receiving yards for a sixth straight season. I'm so grateful Reggie was willing to stay with the Colts. One day, not long after the season ended, Reggie came over and gave me the orange gloves. They're now proudly displayed in my office at home.

Our other rookies on the team delivered some amazing performances as well. Dwayne Allen set a club rookie record for tight ends with 45 receptions. Receiver T.Y. Hilton set a club rookie record with five 100-yard receiving games. Many of the other new guys stepped up and played phenomenal football, regardless of whether or not they broke records.

Our veterans delivered as well. For the fifteenth season in his career, our kicker Adam Vinatieri went over the 100-point mark. Jerrell Freeman had 202 tackles, setting an unofficial club record, and Pat McAfee, the guy who ignited the CHUCKSTRONG movement with a simple tweet, broke his own club record with a gross punting average of 47.9 yards. His career gross punting average rose to 45.4 yards, making him the No. 1 punter in club history. Our defense tied a franchise record by returning four interceptions for touchdowns, two of them by Darius Butler.

Despite the loss to the Ravens, we still managed to exceed everyone's expectations, maybe even our own. We knew we were better than anyone gave us credit for. We knew we were not going to be last in the league or have back-to-back losing seasons. It was simply unacceptable. And when our goals became more challenging because we had to add a fight with cancer to the mix, ultimately it only made us more determined to win.

Adversity will always be part of life. I've said it before, and I'll say it again — circumstances don't define us or determine who we are; they only reveal who we are. We lost the playoff game in Baltimore, but we established a team for all time in Indianapolis.

U

Hey, Chuck — congratulations, my friend. It's great to see you back on the sideline coaching again. I've had a lot of people who know we're friends ask me how you're doing and also ask me how you did it. "Hey, Elks, how did Chuck beat cancer down there in Indy? Some great doctors, right?" Of course you had great doctors. But you and I both know it was more than just the physical treatment that cured you and beat the cancer out of your body.

You had to fight on two different planes. Two different levels, each with its own economy. The one level is the physical plane. And on the physical plane, there's an economy where you trade currency for goods. We all know what money looks like and what we have to pay for tangible purchases like food, clothes, cars, and homes.

However, many people don't always see what takes place in the economy of the second plane — or even recognize the second plane at all. We'll see them talking about football, and they will think that's the only plane. They'll say, "Well, obviously the Indianapolis Colts, they were good," because they could only think of the physical plane. But they don't realize you elevated the team on a different plane.

See, you fought cancer on the physical plane by getting chemo and going into the hospital, taking the medicine, following your doctors' orders. That was the physical front, which is good. But, thank goodness, you also have the second plane, the spiritual plane. See, on that plane you love others. On that plane, there's prayer. You recognize that plane when you said, "Being with the Colts is better than any medicine the doctor could have given me." What you were saying is, "This was medicine on a different plane."

The currency on the physical plane is money. The currency on the spiritual plane is faith. In God's economy, we trade in our faith on the goods. In God's economy, we trade in our faith that our body will be healed, and we trade in our faith on a healthy body.

You can't ignore the physical. For example, if Bruce hadn't been in there with the team teaching the physical skills and plays, then you wouldn't have won. And if your coaches weren't in there teaching the blocking and the tackling, then it would not matter. But you brought the spiritual plane. That's why your leadership goes beyond coaching. You set an example as a spiritual leader, and that's what inspires people. You've heard me say this before, but it's true: Attitudes are contagious — so, is yours worth catching?

If the brightest man alive came to me and gave me scientific evidence that God did not exist and then asked me, "Do you believe now that God doesn't exist?" I would say, "No, I believe God does exist because I've experienced him." The spiritual plane.

When I watched you speak on Christmas Eve and you talked about a child writing you a letter, when I heard you talk on Christmas Eve about the love of your wife, I felt God. When I'm walking down the street and my little girl grabs my hand, I feel him. When someone has forgiven me for something I've done that I wish I hadn't done, all the scientific evidence in the world would not matter because I've experienced him.

For you to continue beating cancer, the economy is faith. For the Colts to keep ascending, the currency is faith. I believed in spite of the evidence, and I watched the evidence change. No one thought your team could be winners — at least not this quickly. Maybe some people doubted your ability to beat cancer — they don't know you. Faith is believing in things you have not seen, and the reward you get if you keep on believing in it is you get to see it.

You believed and you traded in your belief with victory over cancer. That's the currency. Others believed and traded in their faith in supporting you and being there for you, reminding you there's more than just the physical plane. You believed and traded in your faith in a young team that could commit to trust, loyalty, and respect and move to the next level. You believed that a team can catch your attitude and that this makes a difference in the physical plane, as well as in the spiritual.

It's all about faith, Chuck.

Spend your faith.

Give it away.

Faithfully,

Elks

CHAPTER 12

THE 2013 SEASON

Staying in the Hunt

Coaching is a profession of love. You
can't coach people unless you love them.

— Eddie Robinson

Beginning the 2013 season was literally like déjà vu all over again, as Yogi Berra once famously said. It was good to go to work every day, to be back in my normal routines. We take so much for granted when everything in our lives goes along as we expect it to. But in addition to my job still feeling new to me, I had an added layer of appreciation — thanks to what I'd experienced. It wasn't only that my cancer was in remission, but that I was able to beat it with the support and help of our Colts family. More than ever, I was motivated to give our team all I had and to lead the guys to new heights of success.

Some things were different, of course. Once Bruce left for his new job in Phoenix, we had to hire a new offensive coordinator. Our search led us to Pep Hamilton, a rising star in coaching who at the time was at Stanford as their offensive coordinator and quarterbacks coach. Our quarterback Andrew Luck, tight end Coby Fleener, wide receiver Griff Whalen, and strong safety Delano Howell all played for Pep at Stanford and had only the highest praise for both his character and coaching abilities.

In addition to his work at Stanford, Pep spent seven seasons in various coaching roles in the NFL. He served as an offensive coaching assistant and quarterbacks coach with the San Francisco 49ers before becoming quarterbacks coach with the Chicago Bears for four years, where he worked with Jay Cutler.

U

Attending the NFL Scouting Combine and preparing for Draft Day, I was excited to work with Ryan and the rest of our staff to make some key additions to our team. People sometimes ask me what we look for in a player — how we know he'll be a good fit for our program. It's a hard question to answer because there are so many variables. When we look at these prospective players — either free agents or potential draft picks — there's a lot of evaluation that takes place. We look at their body of work at the college level and with another team if they've already played in the league, at their highlights reel and game tapes. We also to go beyond all the facts and stats and determine if these are what we like to call "horseshoe guys."

The horseshoe emblem of the Colts shows seven nails or studs. Each one represents a quality we want in a player/leader for our team — smart, tough, dynamic, physical, character, integrity, and respect. That's what we mean when we say we're looking for a horseshoe guy — guys who play the game the way it was meant to be played. Players who want to be a part of something bigger. Something great.

U

Overall, we were still a young team with many returning players. Even for the guys going into their sophomore year, the past year provided them with more than just one season's worth of experience. Heading into the summer, I felt so grateful all over again to be doing what I love. I was more optimistic than ever — about my health, about our team, and about the future. If we continued to demonstrate the commitment to one another as a team that we had demonstrated in the past season, I knew there was no stopping us.

On June 17, 2013, I was selected by the Pro Football Writers of America (PFWA) as the 2013 George Halas Award winner. This was such an incredible honor. The Halas Award is given to the NFL player, coach, or staff member who overcomes the most adversity to succeed. Although I had overcome adversity that past year, I hadn't done it alone. I gratefully accepted the award, and I thanked everyone who shared it with me — my family; our team; Mr. Irsay; Ryan, Bruce, and all our coaches; our entire organization; our fans; and cancer survivors everywhere. This was truly a team award.

George Halas was a charter member of the Pro Football Hall of Fame, established in 1963 in Canton, Ohio. Halas was a founding father of the NFL through his lifelong association with the Chicago Bears. Over a career spanning forty seasons, he served as a manager, player, promoter, and coach and won 324 games and six NFL titles. I was the forty-fourth Halas Award winner since its inception in 1970, the third NFL head coach to win it, and the fourth member of the Colts to receive this incredible honor.

I had done nothing to deserve winning this award except keep on living and loving the people around me and the game of football. It was a milestone, a special marker that somehow acknowledged the journey we had been through and what we had accomplished as a team, as a family. It was a positive way to move forward from the 2012 season and look ahead to the new season that was about to start.

U

There was something about the uncertainty and unpredictability of life that made me a little apprehensive about going into the new season. Two questions ran through my mind. First, would I remain healthy? As most cancer survivors know, the one-year anniversary is a big deal. If the cancer returns, it's often punctual in coming back a year later.

Second, would players respond to my leading the team the same way they had performed under Bruce during the twelve weeks I was out? I was excited for him in his new position with the Arizona Cardinals and knew we would all enjoy seeing him when we played them in Week 12 that fall. But now I looked forward to coaching an entire season, and I wanted even better results than last season.

Part of the reason I couldn't remain disappointed after our loss to the Ravens was that I knew we had built our foundation on solid rock. We had established something that wasn't going to dry up and blow away in a matter of weeks or months. Our team was committed to building a program for sustained success. We called it "building the monster." We wanted to take our building blocks of athleticism, talent, and skill and bring them to life with our commitment, character, and determination. We wanted to create something that's incredibly strong, resilient in the week-to-week battles of the NFL, and sustainable because of the quality of our relationships with one another.

Looking ahead to the fall, the last thing we wanted was to be a flash in the pan, the emotion-driven team that had achieved a surprising 11 – 5 record in a magical season. Already reporters and bloggers were talking about how there was no way we could repeat the success we had enjoyed in 2012. They said, "The bubble's burst. Chuck's back — and that's great — but now it's back to reality. The magic's gone. They lost their mojo." Their words only made us that much more determined to have a winning season.

Facing cancer forced me to put my beliefs, my faith, and my trust in other people to the test. And we all passed with flying colors, not because we did things differently or floated on waves of powerful emotions. We succeeded because of who we are. It's easy to talk about abstractions like trust, loyalty, and respect and to display them on boards and posters in training rooms and locker rooms. But they are just words, just reminders. If we aren't living them out, each and every day, then when the hard days come, we won't know how to face them.

So while many things had changed between the 2012 and 2013 seasons, the most important things had not. Our commitment to one another was stronger than ever. And once again, it was about to be tested by sixteen opponents with the same goal we had — to win.

U

We shot out of the gate with a win at home against the Raiders in our season opener. But it came at great expense, as we ended up losing two key offensive players. Our second-year tight end Dwayne Allen suffered a hip injury, which we thought would keep him sidelined for only a game or two. But the injury ended up being more serious than first reports indicated, requiring hip surgery that would take Dwayne out for the rest of the season. Then Vick Ballard, our second-year running back who, like Dwayne, had been a critical part of our scoring arsenal the previous year, injured his knee in practice preparing for Week 2's game against the Dolphins.

Injuries are part of the process of playing professional football, but it's never easy to lose guys with the kind of talent, drive, and commitment these two displayed. But you can't make excuses or lose focus by feeling sorry for yourselves. You have to find a way to win — to have other guys step up and to have everyone work together as a team. It's always been about "next man up." Losing someone to injury gives another player an opportunity to fill the role and contribute all he can to our team.

After losing our second game of the season to Miami, we felt even more pressure for the matchup in Week 3 with the San Francisco 49ers. Led by head coach Jim Harbaugh, the brother of my former boss, John Harbaugh, whom Jim had lost to in the previous year's Super Bowl, the 49ers were a great football team. Coming off a road loss to Seattle the previous week, the team under Coach Harbaugh was 7 – 0 in their next game following a loss. Their young, talented quarterback Colin Kaepernick had not lost at home since being named the starter the prior year. Statistically, the odds were against us. The Vegas bookmakers had us as 10-point underdogs.

In addition, there were lots of relational connections and history between our two teams. Andrew, Coby, Griff, and Delano had been coached by Jim Harbaugh at Stanford. Jim had once been the quarterback for the Colts. The media hype was at an all-time high. We knew it would be a huge game, one that would reveal our strengths and weaknesses.

But we were ready for it. We had acquired running back Trent Richardson from Cleveland only days before the game, and he scored a 1-yard touchdown on his first carry as a Colt. During the off-season, we had acquired another running back new to the Colts, former New York Giant Ahmad Bradshaw, and he scored in the last minutes of the game on another 1-yard run. In between, Andrew consistently kept our offensive momentum alive on scoring drives, while our defense held the usually high-scoring Kaepernick to 150 total yards, as he connected on 13 of 27 passes. We intercepted him once and sacked him three times.

Beating the 49ers 27 – 7 built our confidence and reinforced what we knew to be true — we were a great team that could win games and make it to the Super Bowl. This win was a building block, a signature win that would help us continue to build a successful program.

U

We kept winning for a couple more games, beating the Jags in Jacksonville and then taking a close one at home against Seattle. Going into Week 6, we were 4 – 1 as we headed on the road to San Diego. My brother, John, is the defensive coordinator for the Chargers, and it's always great to get to see him when we play each other. He had been a great support during the previous year, even making a trip to Indy to see me during his team's bye week. We hadn't talked much this season, since we were consumed by the attention required by our jobs, so it would be good to see each other after the game.

It was a Monday Night Football game on ESPN, which always brings the national spotlight to that week's game. The Chargers ended up beating us 19 – 9, and we were all disappointed. Don't get me wrong — the Chargers are a great team and played really well that night. It's just that we didn't play our best game. After beating teams like San Francisco and Seattle, I knew we were capable of more. We would have to be. The following week's game loomed on the horizon — a contest against the Denver Broncos.

Not since Brett Favre returned as the quarterback for the Minnesota Vikings to play his former team, the Green Bay Packers, has a game drawn so much hype, attention, and expectations. Peyton Manning would be returning to play football in Indianapolis, this time wearing the blue and orange of the Denver Broncos and not the blue and white of the Colts. To make it really interesting, Peyton was having an exceptional season, one of the best of his career, and the Broncos were undefeated.

In fact, Denver was enjoying a record-breaking, high-scoring season that extended a seventeen-game winning streak from the year before. Everyone thought they looked unbeatable. That perception, coupled with the mixed emotions of Manning's return to our franchise to do battle against a club he had led to numerous wins, division championships, and a Super Bowl win, made our matchup look more like an episode of *Survivor* than a midseason Sunday night football game.

Hosting a former Colts team member, a future Hall of Famer who helped establish the house in which we now hosted him and the Broncos, we were determined to be as welcoming and gracious as we could — and then to play our best game and come away with a win. When Peyton and his team entered the field, we showed a ninety-second tribute video that included some of his most memorable moments as the Colts' quarterback: completing his record-breaking pass to Marvin Harrison for the most touchdowns by a QB-receiver duo, earning the AFC Championship with a comeback win against New England, and winning the Vince Lombardi Trophy at Super Bowl XLI by beating the Chicago Bears. As the crowd gave him a standing ovation, Peyton stopped his warmups and took off his helmet and waved to the cheering fans, visibly emotional as he mouthed "thank you" repeatedly. The mood of the crowd was best summed up by a fan's sign that read, "Thanks, Peyton, But Tonight I'm a Colts Fan!"

The game turned out to be a high-scoring shooting match. Andrew Luck did a fantastic job, completing 21 of 38 passes for 228 total yards, including three touchdowns and no interceptions. The Broncos, however, made mistakes that cost them both time and missed opportunities. Peyton lost a fumble, threw an interception, and suffered four sacks, two of them at the hands of his former teammate Robert Mathis, one of the few remaining players from Manning's time with the Colts.

Denver's kick returner fumbled twice, allowing us to capitalize on one of the recoveries with a touchdown. The Broncos defense was plagued with penalties, especially in the second half. While they stayed in the game until the end, the Broncos coughed up a fourth turnover with only 3:03 remaining that secured our win by a final score of 39 – 33.

U

Like most wins, this one against Denver came with a price. Reggie Wayne tore his right ACL and was going to need season-ending surgery. Our thirteen-year veteran suffered the injury as he reached for a pass from Andrew in the middle of the fourth quarter, and he had to go to the sideline for the remainder of the game. Initial reports from our team doctors were confirmed by an MRI the following day.

As hard as it is to lose any player to injury, this one really stung. You can't easily replace someone like Reggie. This injury broke his record of 189 consecutive games, the most by an active wide receiver. That record reflects his grit and determination, and only an injury of this magnitude could keep him off the field. I encouraged him as best I could, and I made it clear the team and I missed his leadership, his personality, and his humor as much as we missed his athleticism and skill.

"I'll be back," Reggie told me, and I knew it was true. This kind of injury has the potential to end a player's career, especially a veteran of more than a decade. But most players aren't

Reggie Wayne. He has an incredible will, and I know he'll do everything in his power to play football again, even faster and better than what he's done before. As I told a reporter that week, "We'll all put on the orange gloves for Reggie, and we'll help him get through this."

It's what families do.

U

We enjoyed our bye in Week 8, allowing us to rest and prepare for the second half of the season, a task compounded by the loss of Reggie and other key players to injury. In Week 9, we narrowly beat the Houston Texans, 27 – 24 in a game that was eclipsed by the collapse of Texans' head coach Gary Kubiak on the field right at the start of halftime. After going to his knees, he stretched out on the ground as staff and medics quickly gathered around.

The team and I said a prayer for him when we found out, knowing exactly what it's like to lose a coach in the middle of the season. We prayed it would not be something serious. Gary was taken to an area hospital, and we learned later in the week that he had suffered a transient ischemic attack (TIA), a temporary blockage of a blood vessel in the brain that resulted in the kind of dizziness he experienced when he collapsed. Untreated, a TIA can lead to a stroke, but fortunately Gary's blockage was caught early and could be treated.

Defensive coordinator Wade Phillips served as head coach for the second half and almost led the Texans to a victory. But we held on to pull out the win and move our record to 6 – 2.

We weren't so fortunate, however, the following week when St. Louis beat us at Lucas Oil Stadium 38 – 8. We were clearly struggling without Reggie. Andrew Luck continued to find receivers and give it his all. But the season's ups and downs and the injury count were starting to take a toll. And we still had seven games to go.

U

In Week 11, we bounced back in a short week and narrowly beat the Tennessee Titans in Nashville. Coby Fleener had an especially great game, with a career-high eight catches for 107 yards. With this win, we continued our streak of not losing two games in a row.

Next we faced the Arizona Cardinals, now under the head coaching leadership of Bruce Arians. They continued the incredible momentum of the great season they were having by beating us 40 – 11, definitely a disappointment for our team. Bruce didn't have to use any inside knowledge to beat us. Without Reggie Wayne and the other players we'd lost, we remained vulnerable. In our past four games, we had been outscored in the first half 93 – 12. Our offense was stalled and having difficulty finding new ways to start back up.

I told a reporter after the loss to the Cardinals, "There's blood in the water right now. Until we get it fixed, they're going to keep coming at us. It's the same thing week in and week out on both sides of the ball and on special teams. They're going to keep coming at us until we put out the fire."

Despite our struggles, we still led the division in the AFC South, a lead we extended in Week 13 by beating the Titans for a second time. But the three-steps-forward, two-steps-back dance continued when the Cincinnati Bengals beat us 42 – 28 on the road. We just couldn't get things going soon enough. I wasn't the only one getting frustrated with our inability to sustain a winning streak beyond one game. Nonetheless, I tried to practice what I preach and stay focused on the process. One game at a time. Point out the positives, make the necessary corrections, and move on — next play, next game, next day.

U

Thanks to Denver's win over Tennessee, we secured the AFC South title, assuring a wild-card berth in the playoffs. And overcoming our loss to the Bengals the week before, we went on to post a second win over the Houston Texans the following week. We seemed to be stepping up and making the improvements necessary to win consistently, a crucial step if we hoped to make it to the Super Bowl.

In a preview of what would turn out to be the AFC wild-card game, we played the Kansas City Chiefs on the road and won 23 – 7, a huge win against a great team that was having one of its best seasons in decades. With a win at home against the Jaguars, we closed the regular season with a record of 11 – 5, the same as the year before. However, we had gone 6 – 0 against division rivals and had finally found our rhythm in the last three games, outscoring our opponents by a total of 78 – 20.

Like I said, déjà vu all over again. We were going to the playoffs. I had been able to share every minute of every game with our team for the entire season. I couldn't be happier.

U

After all the dozens of notes, emails, and calls that my friend Elks had sent to me over the previous year, I wanted to return the favor. I wanted to be sure he knew just how important his support had been throughout the entire process. Many days, his words of encouragement and insight into our shared faith kept me going. Here's what I wrote to him:

Hey, Elks —

Well, looks like we've come full circle, my friend. We've been blessed with another winning season and are headed to the playoffs. Just thinking of you and wanted to let you know how much I appreciate you and all you've done for me throughout the many years we've been friends, but especially during this past year. Your gift with words, the depth of your faith, and the consistent, heartfelt encouragement sustained me.

I'm still living out the vision, staying in the hunt for the next win, waiting to dance at my daughters' weddings, and looking forward to hoisting the Lombardi Trophy and celebrating with our guys. Whether that's this year or next, or some other year, I don't know. But I can see it, Elks. Thanks to you and the many, many other people who have loved, supported, and carried me through my battle with cancer, I can see the future.

Now I want to give back what I've been given. I want Tina and our daughters and grandkids to know, more than ever, how much I love them and need them in my life. I want our team to know, more than ever, how dedicated I am to them. I want the thousands of boys and girls and men and women fighting for their lives to know they can win. They can beat this bully called cancer.

I want them to know that cancer can take away a lot — your hair, your appetite, your energy, and, yes, sometimes your very life. But cancer cannot take away the love that passes between you and the special people in your life. It can't take away the support and encouragement, the creativity and beauty, the connections and relationships to others who are fighting alongside you. No matter how hard it tries, cancer can never contain the human spirit or diminish the power of faith.

Elks, thank you for everything.

Your buddy,

Chuck

BUILDING A LEGACY

The difference between a successful person
and others is not a lack of strength, not a
lack of knowledge, but rather a lack of will.

—Vince Lombardi

Our game against the Kansas City Chiefs was one for the ages.

At the beginning of the 2013 season, I wanted us to make it clear that last year's winning season was no fluke. We proved that by winning 11 out of 16 games, including wins over both teams that eventually ended up in the Super Bowl, Seattle and Denver. But as we faced playing Kansas City in the AFC wild-card game, we all wanted a win so badly, if for no other reason than to just keep going and play the next game. We wanted to show the world we could go farther than just one game in the postseason. We wanted to go to the Super Bowl, but in the meantime, we had to concentrate on the next game.

As division champs who had already defeated the Chiefs, we had home-field advantage. Everyone was excited, pumped up, and ready to beat KC again and move on to the next round. Not that anyone expected it to be an easy game — *never* assume that in the NFL — but we knew we were capable of beating them.

We stayed with them in the first quarter, trailing by only three points, 10 – 7. But their offense exploded in the second quarter, scoring three touchdowns and leading us at the half, 31 – 10. We even heard a few boos going into the locker room at halftime. This was not going well, to say the least. We were better than this.

So I gave our guys in the locker room the tried-and-true message they had heard so many times before: "There's nothing we can do about the first half — it's over! Let's go out and play Colts football. It's about fundamentals and technique. Blocking, tackling, throwing, and catching — these things never change. Stick to the process. Thirty minutes is all we got. One play at a time; don't judge."

We ended up getting worse before we got better. On his first pass in the third quarter, Andrew threw an interception that was returned to our 18-yard line. Three plays later, the Chiefs were up 38 – 10 — four touchdowns ahead of us. *Four* scores. No time to panic now.

Then something changed. We began to play Colts football. We started to make some plays and get ourselves back in the game.

Andrew had already established himself as a gifted quarterback who could lead a team from behind late in the game to a victory. But his performance was about to take comeback to a whole new level!

We went to a no-huddle offense, and Andrew had permission to fire at will. This allowed us to catch the Chiefs' defense off guard and to begin whittling away at the deficit. With some help from KC's turnovers, by the end of the third quarter, we were back within striking distance, trailing by only 10 points. By the last quarter of the game, Andrew had scored two more touchdowns and recovered a fumble for a touchdown as well. The Chiefs managed to score a field goal, but Andrew found T.Y. on a 64-yard touchdown pass. It was simply *unbelievable*: Colts 45, Chiefs 44 — the final score on the scoreboard.

We overcame the second-largest deficit of any team in an NFL playoff game. Only Buffalo's catch-up comeback of 32 points over Houston in 1993 was larger, and it included the overtime period. We had won the game by one point and would be advancing to play New England in the AFC divisional playoff game. It was almost like we wanted to show just how good we were by contrasting it against how bad we could be.

Like I said, one for the ages.

U

Playing the Patriots on a rainy evening in Foxborough, we knew we had our work cut out for us right out of the gate. Andrew Luck threw an interception that resulted in a LeGarrette Blount touchdown run on New England's first possession. He scored again on their second possession. We finally answered back when Andrew hit LaVon Brazill for a 38-yard touchdown.

But we couldn't stop their ground game. Blount ran for a third touchdown in the second quarter, while we added a Vinatieri field goal. I thought the tide might be turning right before the half when a bad snap by the Patriots sailed over punter Ryan Allen's head, resulting in a safety. Going into the locker room, we trailed 21 – 12. Not a great situation, but considering what we'd experienced the week before, doable.

The second half became a soggy mess of mistakes and missed opportunities. Blount ran for a fourth touchdown, this one for 73 yards, propelling him to a total of 166 yards and tying a playoff record. Our guys tried to keep us in it, but we couldn't overcome our turnovers. By the time the game ended, we had lost 43 – 22, sending the Patriots to take on the Denver Broncos in the AFC Championship game.

It wasn't the way we wanted to end the season, especially after our huge comeback win the week before. But this kind of game is just as much a part of the process as that dramatic win against the Chiefs. Whether we win or lose, we have to stay focused on getting better and playing our next game. We had come farther this season, and I was proud of our team. We have a rock-solid foundation for the 2014 season.

I can already see us with the Lombardi Trophy. We've got some work to do between now and then. But never count us out.

We love a challenge!

U

In the late 1400s in Nuremberg, Germany, two brothers, Albrecht and Albert, grew up wanting to be artists. They came from a very large family of more than a dozen siblings, and their father was a goldsmith. Although their family was relatively well-off by the standards of that day, their parents could not afford to send both of them to study art. So as the brothers grew older, Albert told his brother, "Albrecht, I want you to go and study to be an artist. You have an amazing talent, and I know you will draw and paint many beautiful works. I'm going to work in order to pay for your studies."

"How? What will you do?" asked his younger brother.

"I'll work in the mines if I have to," Albert said. "Your talent is so great that I'll do whatever it takes to see it come to fruition."

So at the age of about fifteen, Albrecht left his family home to study as the apprentice of a great artist of their day, Michael Wolgemut. After his apprenticeship, he traveled to other places in Europe, including Italy, which was the center of the renaissance taking place in art. From the beginning, Albrecht's talent was recognized by teachers and critics alike. All who saw his work couldn't believe how good he was. His gift with pencil, ink, woodcuts, and paint emerged in every piece he created.

After several years, Albrecht returned home to Nuremberg. When he came home, his father threw him a feast for everything he had done and to show how proud they were of him. And where had his brother Albert been all this time? Down in the mines, grinding away so that Albrecht could fulfill his dream. Albert was serving a dream bigger than himself.

Midway through the feast, Albrecht got up to make a toast to his brother. With his voice trembling with emotion, Albrecht toasted his brother and thanked him for his sacrifice. He thanked him for going down in that mine for him so that Albrecht could go out and fulfill his dream. Albrecht concluded by saying, "For your great gift of service, Albert, I am now going to go down in the mine so *you* can go to art school and fulfill *your* dream."

Albert got up, tears in his eyes, and thanked his brother for the gesture. Then he said, "Brother, look at my hands." He held them up for all to see. His hands were worn, broken, calloused. There was no way he could go off to art school and do anything because his hands were in such terrible shape. He couldn't even hold a pencil or paintbrush.

So Albrecht became determined to draw and paint enough for the both of them. He continued his career and left dozens of beautiful works, many of them that are on display in churches. However, he is probably best known for a sketch he did as part of a three-piece panel in a church. The sketch shows two hands clasped in prayer. These hands are beautifully drawn and rich in detail, with long, tapered fingers and prominent veins. Albrecht wanted to honor his brother, and so he powerfully and poignantly captured the sacrifice Albert had made for him in the rough-hewn beauty of this drawing known simply as *Praying Hands*.

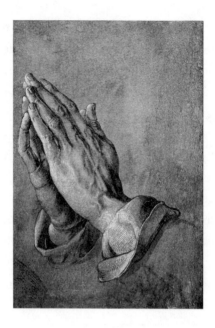

∪

Although there are various versions with unknown sources of this story, this is the version I like to share at the beginning of each season and ask our players, our staff, and our coaches a series of simple questions: Would you go down in the mine for a loved one? Would you go down in the mine for a sick child? Would you go down in the mine for your coworker? Would you go down in the mine for a family member? For somebody who's hurting? To fulfill someone else's dream?

Our guys get it. They understand the enormous sacrifice that Albert made so his brother's art could come to life and be enjoyed by countless future generations. These guys know what it means to give themselves up for the good of the team. They go down in the mine and pull out a win in overtime. They stretch a little farther, jump a little higher, push a little harder to make plays happen so the team can win.

Regardless of the position they play, they all buy in to the same level of sacrifice. They have faith in one another and in the sacrifices of time, energy, strength, and emotional intensity they're investing. They want to pay the price to be part of something bigger than themselves.

What is faith? Faith is believing in something you can't see. Right now we can't see a cure for cancer, not literally in front of us. But the vision is there, and countless teams of individuals — doctors and nurses, scientists and researchers — are living the vision. They see a day in the not-so-distant future when we will live in a cancer-free world. As this book goes to press, the CHUCKSTRONG campaign has raised almost two million dollars in the fight against cancer. We just have to keep living the vision and grinding away for the victory — one play at a time, one day at a time.

This is the battle we're all called to fight. Life takes us out of the game, and suddenly we're sidelined. For me, it was the fight against cancer; for our team, it was the fight to make it to the playoffs. But this same process of perseverance can help you face whatever impossible challenge you might be facing. No matter how great the odds seem that are stacked against you, it's never too late to put hope in action. You just have to take life as it comes, doing the next thing and then the next. Never be afraid to ask for help and to accept the support you're given. Give it everything you've got, and trust God for the outcome.

Remember, your condition does not determine your position. You must understand your condition but focus on your positive position — to hope, to love, to serve. YOU WILL! YOU CAN! YOU MUST! YOU HAVE NO CHOICE. BY ANY MEANS NECESSARY. YOU WILL OVERCOME.

ACKNOWLEDGMENTS

We gratefully acknowledge the contributions of the many people who have made this book possible.

The Colts family. Team owner Jim Irsay; his daughters, Carlie, Casey, Kalen; and the rest of their family. Ryan Grigson, Pete Ward, Dan Emerson, Bruce Arians. The Colts' coaching, training, and medical staffs; the players; the people in marketing and sales and in the personnel department. The entire Colts organization and their families. And all of the coaches and players we've been fortunate to work with over the years.

Dr. Cripe and Mimi, Stacey Dye, and all the great doctors, nurses, and caregivers at IU Simon Cancer Center. All the people who serve and work in research in the battle against cancer — *Never ever give up!* All of the fine people and fans in the great city of Indianapolis and state of Indiana. All those who shared their stories, young and old. To Cory and Mickey. To everybody who makes the CHUCKSTRONG Foundation such a success.

David Morris, John Sloan, Dirk Buursma, Alicia Kasen, Heather Adams, Kim Tanner, Sarah Johnson, Curt Diepenhorst, and all the people at Zondervan. For the contributions of Dudley Delffs, Kevin Elko, Bob Shook, and the guys at REP 1 Sports.

We especially want to thank our families. The Tollners: wife, Lisa, and children, Justin, Cassidy and Jordan. Parents Ted and Barbara Tollner. The Paganos: wife, Tina, and children, Tara (husband, Kenny, and children, Avery, Addie, and Zoey), Taylor, and Tori. Parents Sam and Diana Pagano and the Heffner family.

Acknowledgment isn't a strong enough word to express the love and appreciation for those who made these pages the story it is. Many of you are not even mentioned by name. You know who you are. Our gratitude knows no bounds. Thank you!

INDIANAPOLIS COLTS ROSTER

Kris Adams	Tim Fugger	Kyle Miller
Mario Addison	Josh Gordy	Fili Moala
James Aiono	Marshay Green	Mewelde Moore
Dwayne Allen	Lawrence Guy	Drake Nevis
Justin Anderson	Chandler Harnish	Mike Newton
Pat Angerer	Mario Harvey	Seth Olsen
Donnie Avery	Justin Hickman	Matt Overton
Vick Ballard	Tony Hills	Nathan Palmer
Antoine Bethea	T.Y. Hilton	Mike Person
LaVon Brazill	Delano Howell	Jerraud Powers
Donald Brown	Jerry Hughes	Cory Redding
Jerry Brown	Ben Ijalana	Joe Reitz
Mario Brown	Antonio Johnson	Jabin Sambrano
Sergio Brown	Dominique Jones	Samson Satele
Darius Butler	Winston Justice	Weslye Saunders
Delone Carter	Deji Karim	A.Q. Shipley
Anthony Castonzo	Brandon King	Bradley Sowell
Josh Chapman	Justin King	Drew Stanton
Austin Collie	Joe Lefeged	Martin Tevaseu
Kavell Conner	Korey Lindsey	Cassius Vaughn
Vontae Davis	Jeff Linkenbach	Adam Vinatieri
Antonio Dixon	Andrew Luck	Reggie Wayne
A.J. Edds	Scott Lutrus	Jamaal Westerman
Trai Essex	Ricardo Mathews	Griff Whalen
Coby Fleener	Robert Mathis	Teddy Williams
Moise Fokou	Pat McAfee	Tom Zbikowski
Jerrell Freeman	Mike McGlynn	
Dwight Freeney	Brandon McKinney	

INDIANAPOLIS COLTS
COACHING STAFF

Chuck Pagano	Gary Emanuel
Bruce Arians	Jeff FitzGerald
Greg Manusky	Mike Gillhamer
Clyde Christensen	Roy Anderson
David Walker	Brad White
Charlie Williams	Marwan Maalouf
Alfredo Roberts	Brant Boyer
Harold Goodwin	Roger Marandino
Joe Gilbert	Richard Howell
Frank Giufre	James Betcher

INDIANAPOLIS COLTS SCHEDULE

PRESEASON

Sunday, August 12	vs. St. Louis	W, 38–3
Sunday, August 19	at Pittsburgh	L, 26–24
Saturday, August 25	at Washington	L, 30–17
Thursday, August 30	vs. Cincinnati	W, 20–16

REGULAR SEASON

Sunday, September 9	at Chicago	L, 41–21
Sunday, September 16	vs. Minnesota	W, 23–20
Sunday, September 23	vs. Jacksonville	L, 22–17
Sunday, September 30	Bye Week	
Sunday, October 7	vs. Green Bay	W, 30–27
Sunday, October 14	at New York	L, 35–9
Sunday, October 21	vs. Cleveland	W, 17–13
Sunday, October 28	at Tennessee	W, 19–13 OT
Sunday, November 4	vs. Miami	W, 23–20
Thursday, November 8	at Jacksonville	W, 27–10
Sunday, November 18	at New England	L, 59–24
Sunday, November 25	vs. Buffalo	W, 20–13
Sunday, December 2	at Detroit	W, 35–33
Sunday, December 9	vs. Tennessee	W, 27–23
Sunday, December 16	at Houston	L, 29–17
Sunday, December 23	at Kansas City	W, 20–13
Sunday, December 30	vs. Houston	W, 28–16

POSTSEASON
Wild-Card Round

Sunday, January 6	at Baltimore	L, 24–9

INDIANAPOLIS COLTS SCHEDULE

PRESEASON

Sunday, August 11	vs. Buffalo	L, 44–20
Sunday, August 18	at New York	W, 20–12
Saturday, August 24	vs. Cleveland	W, 27–6
Thursday, August 29	at Cincinnati	L, 27–10

REGULAR SEASON

Sunday, September 8,	vs. Oakland	W, 21–17
Sunday, September 15	vs. Miami	L, 24–20
Sunday, September 22	at San Francisco	W, 27–7
Sunday, September 29	at Jacksonville	W, 37–3
Sunday, October 6	vs. Seattle	W, 34–28
Monday, October 14	at San Diego	L, 19–9
Sunday, October 20	vs. Denver	W, 39–33
Sunday, October 27	Bye Week	
Sunday, November 3	at Houston	W, 27–24
Sunday, November 10	vs. St. Louis	L, 38–8
Thursday, November 14	at Tennessee	W, 30–27
Sunday, November 24	at Arizona	L, 40–11
Sunday, December 1	vs. Tennessee	W, 22–14
Sunday, December 8	at Cincinnati	L, 42–28
Sunday, December 15	vs. Houston	W, 25–3
Sunday, December 22	at Kansas City	W, 23–7
Sunday, December 29	vs. Jacksonville	W, 30–10

POSTSEASON

Wild-Card Round

Sunday, January 4	vs. Kansas City	W, 45–44

Divisional Round

Saturday, January 10	at New England	L, 43–22

ABOUT COACH PAGANO

Chuck Pagano's 2012 season proved to be one of the most inspirational stories in NFL history. Named head coach of the Indianapolis Colts on January 25, 2012, Pagano was forced to take a leave of absence just three games into the season after being diagnosed with acute promyelocytic leukemia, a curable form of the disease, which is a cancer of the blood and bone marrow cells.

The news shocked not only the Colts' organization, but the city of Indianapolis and people all over the country as well. With a 1 – 2 record, the Colts were without their leader in the midst of a transition that had started to take shape in the off-season. Those who expected the Colts to falter didn't understand the principles on which Pagano built his squad. Terms like *trust, loyalty, respect,* and *team* resonate throughout the Indiana Farm Bureau Football Center and are applied when the Colts take to the gridiron on Sundays.

When Pagano hired Bruce Arians as the team's offensive coordinator, he knew exactly what kind of coach and person would be directing the Colts' offense. Pagano and Arians coached together for the Cleveland Browns (2001 – 2003) and went toe-to-toe in an AFC North Division rivalry when Arians served as the offensive coordinator for the Pittsburgh

Steelers and Pagano held the position of defensive coordinator for the Baltimore Ravens. Pagano also knew Arians would lead the team based on the foundation currently in place while continuing to develop the groundwork and expectations that Pagano established during his first months at the helm.

Now serving as the team's interim head coach, Arians and the Colts defied the odds and rallied to a 9 – 3 record. During that time frame, Indianapolis secured a playoff berth and accomplished one of their primary goals — extending the season for Coach Pagano. Some of the victories during Arians's term included a comeback win against Green Bay (Week 5) after trailing by 18 points, an overtime victory on the road at Tennessee (Week 8), and a last-second victory in Detroit (Week 13). In all, the Colts posted a 9 – 1 record in one-possession games in 2012, including winning their last eight.

As much as Chuck Pagano inspired the 2012 Colts, the team did just the same for their ailing head coach. From his hospital bed, Pagano was in constant communication with the coaching staff and players. He analyzed practices while continuing to game-plan schemes. Along the way, Pagano continued to make his presence felt. After the team's Week 9 victory against Miami, the head coach gave a moving postgame speech to the contingent in the locker room.

"I've got circumstances," Pagano told the team in the locker room. "You guys understand it; I understand it. It's already beat [referring to the leukemia]. It's already beat. My vision that I'm living is to see two more daughters get married, dance at their weddings, and then hoist that Lombardi Trophy several times."

Pagano made another return three weeks later during the team's win against Buffalo, when he appeared in owner and

CEO Jim Irsay's suite while saluting the crowd. Pagano received a rousing ovation from Colts fans in attendance.

As the season took shape, the Colts' organization and Indianapolis community rallied behind their head coach. The CHUCKSTRONG movement was well under way. CHUCK-STRONG T-shirts and wristbands were offered for sale, with proceeds going to leukemia research. The team established a collection benefiting leukemia research at their October 21 game against Cleveland and also held a blood drive. Several Colts players shaved their heads in support of their head coach, while thousands in the Indianapolis community followed suit. Two Colts cheerleaders even raised $10,000 for leukemia research, as they agreed to have their heads shaved during the team's November 25 contest against Buffalo.

As the regular season came to an end, the culmination of Arians's stretch as interim head coach concluded with the team's playoff-clinching victory at Kansas City (Week 16). The stage was set for Pagano to return after missing twelve weeks of action. In the week leading up to the game, Pagano addressed the media regarding his return.

"It's really great to be back," said Pagano. "Like a kid in a candy store, I get to come and be around the guys again. Do what I love to do and what I've done my whole life. Obviously we don't ever want to take anything for granted. I want you to know — our entire country to know and everybody in the NFL who was so kind, generous, loving, and supportive — what a privilege it is to coach in the National Football League. It is the greatest sport in the world, and I feel very honored."

Division rival Houston visited Lucas Oil Stadium in the regular season finale in hopes of clinching the AFC's No. 1

seed in the playoffs. The Colts were not to be deterred, however, as the team corralled the emotion in Pagano's return and earned a 28 – 16 win to finish the regular season with an 11 – 5 record. The real victory, however, was the return of a healthy Chuck Pagano. It was a day the Colts' organization and fans will remember for generations.

Indianapolis's playoff run ended earlier than the team had wished after falling to the eventual Super Bowl XLVII champion Baltimore Ravens in an AFC wild-card playoff contest. What was not lost were the numerous team and individual milestones that the Colts established in a season carrying low expectations. Most notably, the 11 – 5 record was a 9-win improvement from the 2011 campaign, which tied for the third largest one-year turnaround in NFL history. The Colts also registered their twelfth 10-plus win season in the past fourteen years, which is the most of any NFL team since 1999. Pagano and Arians were honored together by the Maxwell Football Club as the recipients of the 24th Annual Earle "Greasy" Neale Award for Professional Coach of the Year. The two also garnered AFC Coach of the Year honors as winners of the annual NFL 101 Awards. Pagano was selected by the Pro Football Writers of America (PFWA) as the winner of the 2013 George Halas Award, given to an NFL player, coach, or staff member who overcame the most adversity to succeed. Each year, the Fritz Pollard Alliance Foundation recognizes individuals who make a difference in diversity and inclusion at an annual awards banquet. In February 2013, Pagano received the foundation's Game Ball Award for the differences he has made to level the playing field in the NFL for minorities.

The 2013 season marked Pagano's thirtieth year of coaching and twelfth season in the NFL. Prior to joining the Colts, he spent four seasons with the Baltimore Ravens and the last (2011) as the team's defensive coordinator.

In 2011, Pagano's defensive unit finished third in the NFL in total defense (288.9 ypg), second against the run (92.6 ypg), and fourth against the pass (196.3 ypg) on their way to an appearance in the AFC Championship Game. The Ravens also led the league in forced fumbles (21) and had the third-most sacks in the NFL (48.0), including a franchise record-tying 9.0 in Week 12 against San Francisco.

Pagano served as the Ravens' secondary coach for three seasons (2008 – 2010) before taking the reins as defensive coordinator. As the team's secondary coach, he led a defensive backfield that had to adjust to a number of injuries, including a significant loss of seven-time Pro Bowl safety Ed Reed, who started the 2010 campaign on the Physically Unable to Perform (PUP) list. Even after missing the first six games, Reed still led the league with 8 interceptions in only 10 games.

In Pagano's first season with the Ravens (2008), the team led the NFL with 26 interceptions, including Ed Reed's NFL-high 9 picks. Reed, the league's only unanimous (50 votes) All-Pro in 2008, was also coached by Pagano at the University of Miami. Pagano's secondary also ranked second against the pass (179.7 ypg), as the defense ranked No. 2 overall in the league, a drastic improvement from a No. 20 finish in 2007.

In his four seasons in Baltimore, Pagano's defenses allowed the second-fewest points per game (16.3) and the second-fewest net yards (292.3) in the NFL. The Ravens also ranked third in the NFL in scoring defense during that span.

Pagano posted a one-year stint as the defensive coordinator at North Carolina (2007), where he rejoined Butch Davis from previous stops with the Cleveland Browns and Miami

Hurricanes. Under Pagano, the defense improved from 92nd in the nation in 2006 to 35th in 2007.

Prior to UNC, Pagano spent two seasons (2005 – 06) as the defensive backs coach of the Oakland Raiders. In 2006, the Raiders led the NFL in pass defense, allowing just 150.8 yards per game, and ranked third in total defense, surrendering only 284.8 yards per contest. Cornerback Nnamdi Asomugha ranked third in the NFL with eight interceptions in 2006.

From 2001 – 04, Pagano coached the Cleveland secondary under then-head coach Butch Davis. In 2003, the defensive backs helped the Browns tie the franchise record for the fewest passing touchdowns allowed in a season with 13. Under Pagano's guidance in 2001, Cleveland accounted for 28 of the team's NFL-leading and team-record 33 interceptions. That season, rookie cornerback Anthony Henry led the NFL with 10 picks.

Pagano returned to the University of Miami (1995 – 2000) for his second stint at the school, coaching the Hurricanes' secondary as well as serving as special teams coordinator. He coached four NFL first-round defensive backs: Ed Reed (Ravens, 24th – 2002), Phillip Buchanon (Raiders, 17th – 2002), Duane Starks (Ravens, 10th – 1998), and Mike Rumph (49ers, 27th – 2002). During Pagano's second tenure in Miami, the Hurricanes blocked 39 kicks in 59 games. In 2000, the secondary was named the nation's best by Football News. His special teams unit also set a school record in 1996 with 12 blocked kicks.

Pagano started his coaching career as a graduate assistant at Southern California (1984 – 85) before taking the same role at the University of Miami (1986). In 1987, he started a two-year stint at Boise State, where he coached outside linebackers. Pagano then spent one season (1989) at East Carolina, coaching the secondary, before moving to UNLV, where he led the secondary (1990) and eventually was named defensive coordinator in 1991. In 1992, Pagano returned to East Carolina, coaching the secondary and outside linebackers for three seasons (1992 – 94).

Collegiately, Pagano was a four-year letterman and two-year starter at strong safety for the University of Wyoming, from which he graduated with a degree in marketing in 1984.

Pagano was a four-year letterman and two-year starter at strong safety at Fairview (Boulder, Colorado) High School. His brother, John, is the Chargers' defensive coordinator and former defensive assistant for the Colts from 1998 – 2001.

Chuck and his wife, Tina, have three daughters, Tara, Taylor, and Tori, and three granddaughters, Avery, Addison, and Zoey.

COACHING CAREER

1984 – 1985 Southern California, Graduate Assistant
1986 University of Miami, Graduate Assistant
1987 – 1988 Boise State, Outside Linebackers
1989 East Carolina, Secondary
1990 – 1991 University of Nevada, Las Vegas (UNLV), Defensive Coordinator/Secondary
1992 – 1994 East Carolina, Secondary/Outside Linebackers
1995 – 2000 University of Miami, Secondary/Special Teams
2001 – 2004 Cleveland Browns, Secondary
2005 – 2006 Oakland Raiders, Defensive Backs
2007 North Carolina, Defensive Coordinator
2008 – 2010 Baltimore Ravens, Secondary
2011 Baltimore Ravens, Defensive Coordinator
2012 – 2013 Indianapolis Colts, Head Coach

Bio courtesy of Indianapolis Colts

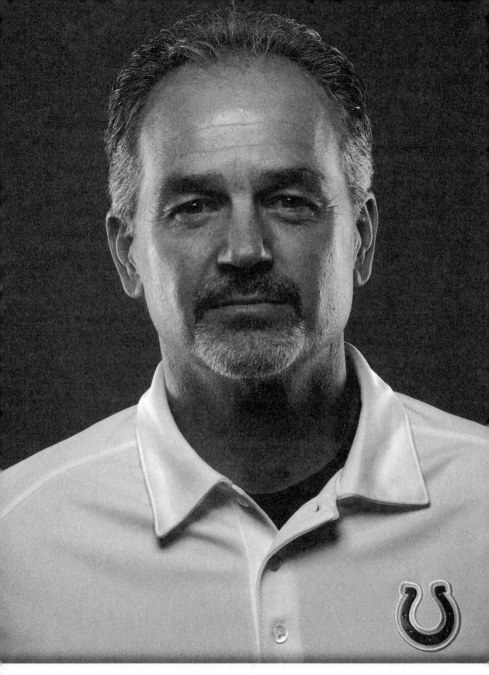

CHUCKSTRONG

To learn more about the CHUCKSTRONG effort or to donate online, go to www.colts.com/Chuckstrong.
All proceeds benefit the IU Simon Cancer Center for cancer research, Riley Hospital for Children, and other charities.